Praise for *When Sk*

"Full of bravery, wisdom, and insight, *When Skies Are Gray* is a tender retelling of resilience. While every reader may not know the loss of a child, Lindsey's words offer something to us all."

—RACHEL LEWIS,
author of *Unexpecting: Real Talk on Pregnancy Loss*

"Lindsey Henke's debut memoir is a beautiful meditation on loss, love, marriage, and family. *When Skies Are Gray* is full of heartbreak, of course, but it is also full of tenderness and hope. Lindsey writes with humor and grace, and her story, ultimately, connects, humanizes, and heals. This is a lovely, much-needed book!"

—KATE HOPPER,
author of *Ready for Air* and *Use Your Words*

"Through *When Skies Are Gray*, Lindsey cracks wide open the stigma that parental grief and bereavement are topics to be avoided in the 'mommy-verse.' The reality is, not every mother leaves the maternity ward with a healthy newborn. But through Lindsey's words, you'll find there is beauty in talking about the sad stories too."

—JANE CHERTOFF,
former editor of *Pregnancy & Newborn* magazine

"A wholehearted, accessible memoir that expresses the depths of grief around stillbirth, along with the possibility of renewal."

—EMMA NADLER, psychotherapist
and author of *The Unlikely Village of Eden: A Memoir*

"Through raw and authentic storytelling, Henke skillfully presents the interplay of grief, joy, and the resilience of the human spirit. A beacon of hope in the literature of grief, this memoir not only breaks your heart but also mends it, teaching us that even amidst the most profound loss, love can find us."

—ALEXA BIGWARFE, author of *Sunshine After the Storm: A Survival Guide for the Grieving Mother*

"Deeply moving, *When Skies Are Gray* is a testament to the fierce power of a parent's love—a force unbreakable even in death. Lindsey Henke's candid account of loss, despair, hope, and healing should be required reading for the newly bereft."

—SAMANTHA DURANTE BANERJEE, founder and executive director of PUSH for Empowered Pregnancy

"As both a therapist and a mother, Lindsey has a unique perspective on grief and loss that is invaluable. Reading of her journey through pregnancy, motherhood, and grief, we're given a window into the soul of a bereaved mother."

—AMANDA ROSS-WHITE, author of *Joy at the End of the Rainbow: A Guide to Pregnancy After a Loss*

"*When Skies Are Gray* is an invaluable companion and essential memoir for bereaved parents on the unpredictable path of motherhood."

—ALEXIS MARIE CHUTE, author of *Expecting Sunshine: A Journey of Grief, Healing, and Pregnancy After Loss*

"*When Skies Are Gray* gracefully balances love, grief, joy, and the intimate connection of mother and child. Lindsey's memoir remarkably encapsulates navigating a life one never would've chosen while simultaneously demonstrating the beauty that remains."

—AMIE LANDS, author of *Navigating the Unknown, Our Only Time, Perfectly Imperfect Family,* and the Tending to Your Heart series

"With candor, Lindsey Henke takes us on a journey of joy and grief, showing us how life, and particularly motherhood, is often lived between the two."

—JENNY ALBERS, author of *Courageously Expecting: 30 Days of Encouragement for Pregnancy After Loss*

"Written with grace and vivid descriptions of the journey of the loss of her child, Henke shares her climb back into a life that will never be the same alongside her continued bond and attachment to her daughter, Nora. This book can provide helpful insight to health care providers' understanding of parental grief."

—JOANN O'LEARY, PhD, prenatal parent-infant specialist and coauthor of *Meeting the Needs of Parents Pregnant and Parenting After Perinatal Loss*

"Bereaved parents reading this memoir and those who have not experienced this loss personally will find this story illuminating, while also learning strategies for navigating life and pregnancy after loss."

—KILEY KREKORIAN HANISH, founder of Return to Zero Center for Healing

"This book is a must-read and a must-gift for anyone who has suffered loss or has loved someone who has."

—GALIT BREEN, codirector of Listen to Your Mother Twin Cities

WHEN
SKIES
ARE
GRAY

WHEN

a grieving

SKIES

mother's

ARE

lullaby

GRAY

Lindsey M. Henke

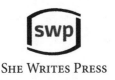

SHE WRITES PRESS

Published 2024
Printed in the United States of America

Print ISBN: 978-1-64742-630-9
E-ISBN: 978-1-64742-631-6
Library of Congress Control Number: 2023919348

For information, address:
She Writes Press
1569 Solano Ave #546
Berkeley, CA 94707

Interior design and typeset by Katherine Lloyd, The DESK

She Writes Press is a division of SparkPoint Studio, LLC.

For my children.

When the world is dark, we seek the light.

You have always been mine.

—Mom

AUTHOR'S NOTES

A note on privacy:

This story has changed names and details to respect loved ones, fellow bereaved parents, and clients' privacy.

A note on memory:

I've shared my truth within this memoir, but anyone who has experienced the fog of grief will understand how our memories often become clouded by our heartache.

A note on terminology:

As a social work practitioner, I believe in the value that an individual is the expert of their own lived experience. Therefore, when referring to myself in therapy and those I am grateful to have had the privilege to provide therapy to, I use the term "client" throughout this book.

A GRIEVING MOTHER'S LULLABY

Through the womb was the only way I ever knew my first child, Nora, who died before she was born. Silent and still, she slipped briefly into this world and out on a cold December evening in 2012. Death stole my daughter from me as I slept in winter's early hours of darkness and left me alone in the deafening blackness of my sorrow, when after nine months of a perfect pregnancy, I went into labor only to be told, "I'm sorry . . . there's no heartbeat."

Death took not only my child but also our future memories yet to be made, like the intonation of love in my murmur of her name she would never hear, and I am left to wonder on what note she would have carried her cry. We were denied the lifetime of nights I had imagined swaying her to sleep with a lullaby.

The grief that lives on in a mother's heart after the stillbirth of her baby is like lyrics to a lullaby, for a lullaby can also be a lament. Frederico Garcia Lorca, a poet in the 1920s, studied Spanish lullabies and noticed a "depth of sadness" in these songs as a mother vocalized her intense love and fear for her child through lyrics and rhythm. Lorca theorized that the function of the lullaby was not only to soothe the baby but also the new mother, serving as a type of therapy for her.[1]

As a young psychotherapist when pregnant with Nora, I'm ashamed to admit I did not go to much therapy before she died. But in the depths of my mourning, finding myself broken and bawling on an empty nursery floor with no baby in my arms to sing my lament to, I turned to trying out therapy techniques I had learned in my few short years of practice on my injured psyche and soul. This led me to create a blog about my grief in the weeks that followed my daughter's death, as well as going to actual therapy to help me find the words to match the notes of my unsung lullaby.

I learned the lyrics to this song slowly over the months and years after Nora's death. During weekly therapy sessions, and through daily blogging, I found the sometimes sweet, often sad lyrics to our shared song: a combination of both a lullaby and a lament, referred to as lullaments.

Lullaments are musical expressions of birth and death, grief and joy, fear and hope, love, and loss—ballads epitomizing a universal truth that life cannot be lived without holding both pleasure and pain within the same sigh.[2]

This may be why these sometimes sad, sometimes joyful tunes—that often hold both emotions—possess a tranquil, hypnotic tone within their rhythm as they dance between the extremes. Like how, years later, I'm still hypnotized by the love left within me for my first daughter, who never heard a hummed note of her mother's tune but was the one who started the song within my heart now sung to her siblings as they fall asleep.

This book is the lullaby I never got to sing to the child that made me a mother. It's the lament I could not leave unsung. It's the lullament of the bereaved mother.

present

"The other night dear, as I lay sleeping
I dreamed I held you in my arms . . ."

—*Jimmie Davies, "You Are My Sunshine"*

I'LL ALWAYS WONDER WHO YOU WOULD HAVE BEEN

"Mama, tell me a story," I imagine her saying as we cuddled, sinking into the pillows side by side next to each other in her room before bed. The glow-in-the-dark stars illuminate the ceiling, and I take in her beauty by the pinkish hue from the salt lamp nightlight. Her long feathery dark hair, like her father's, brushes across the tops of her bony shoulders. I envision her eyes as greenish brown, like her sister's and brother's. At the imagined age of four, I can almost see her growing from the silent and still shell of the baby I held in my arms into a toddler, then a big kid, which she would be calling herself by now since she is my first out of three.

"What story would you like?" I imagine asking as she hugs her favorite toy close to her chest. I picture it as a tattered stuffed elephant worn with time and love, the first gift she received from her aunt Kristi, my sister, before she was stillborn. I watch her give him kisses as I study my daughter, pondering what lullaby she would like to hear.

"Tell me our love story," she finally replies with wide eyes full of wonder, as if it's her most favorite story of all.

Leaning in to stroke her brown, earthy-smelling hair once more, I smile, snuggling deeper under the heavy handprint quilt that her grandmother made. I take a moment to think about where to start. I recall the time when our paths first crossed but then focus on the imagined present, where I can feel her body next to mine, alive—like she was when we were one. And with this wish, my lullaby begins.

Once upon a time . . .

before

"You are my sunshine. My only sunshine . . ."

—*Jimmie Davies, "You Are My Sunshine"*

chapter 1

HAPPILY,
EVER AFTER

Before she was born, I called for her. It's like I conjured her out of the air. Unable to fall asleep next to my husband Nick on a cold dark December night, in our one-bedroom condo, a few months after our marriage, I whispered my request aloud. I asked the gods, the winds, and the heavens I didn't believe in to bring me a child.

By early summer, as I sat in my new office in the therapist chair across from the client couch where I provided counseling for those struggling with addiction, I felt her move. At first, she moved like a butterfly in water, softly batting her wings together to push the amniotic fluid back and forth like ripples turned to waves washing upon the shores of my skin from the inside. Over the weeks, her wing flaps became acrobatic rolls that made my uterus her flying trapeze, and then months later, by late autumn, had evolved into the jabs and kicks of a miniature karate kid. She was always moving, sometimes small, sometimes strong, but all the time persistently present.

Forty weeks pregnant on Christmas Day, I felt her kick again. I placed my hand on my watermelon-sized belly to focus on her movement. Like clockwork, a kick, a jab, then a pause, and finally a slight roll. She moved within me as my eyes drifted to the sliding glass door that opened to our deck, where snow had piled inches high on its railing of our new, two-story suburban home.

The cold scene outside caused me to crawl closer to my husband under the covers of the bed, where our furry black-and-white Shih Tzu, Georgie, made us even warmer by nuzzling onto our feet. Nick immersed himself in the pages of *The Black Swan: The Impact of the Highly Improbable,* one of the many books on his nightstand about philosophy, history, or military strategy, while I took an afternoon nap with my head in his lap. Closing my eyes, I let out a contented exhale, happy with our decision to spend the holiday in our new home in Minnesota instead of heading back to the houses where we had grown up, in opposite neighboring states. We enjoyed the solitude of our last days as a couple before the silence of our childless world would soon be broken by the bustling sounds of bringing home a baby. Or so we believed.

That short winter's day quickly turned into an early dusk with snow mounting outside the window. The previous spring, rains had welcomed us into our newly purchased home and brought with them not just the smell of April flowers, but also a positive plus sign on a pregnancy test. *I'm not ready for this*, I thought as our baby moved once more, and I wondered where the last nine months had gone.

Struggling to sit up next to Nick, I awkwardly positioned myself to face him. My huge belly covered in maternity pajamas rested on my crisscrossed legs. "Are you happy?" I asked earnestly.

Looking up from the page he was reading, Nick collapsed his hardcover book into his lap. His greenish-brown eyes met mine before he replied with his answer I already knew, as Nick was dependable and predictable to the point of bordering on boring, but in a good way.

"I'm the happiest I've ever been," he answered, wrinkling his prominent nose with his smile. Reaching for my middle, he placed his hand on my belly and brought his bristly face to my stomach. His stubble scratched my skin as he spoke sweetly to our child inside. "We can't wait to meet you." He whispered softly as if singing a baby to sleep, "You can come out anytime now."

I brushed my hand through his full head of soft black hair, kept short and clean for his job as a naval intelligence officer. With his head lying in the place between my breasts and belly full with our baby, I was calm, which was out of character for me. I let myself settle into a state of momentary ease, twirling his fine strands through my fingers, as I eavesdropped on the start of what I imagined to be one of many conversations between a father and daughter.

Nick was right. We were happy. We had been from the beginning. Our love story, like so many others in the late 2000s, started online. My tagline was, "A little salty but mostly sweet." His was, "Looking for an adventure," which was exactly what my twenty-five-year-old self was seeking at the time.

Our first date was at one of the most unromantic places in Minnesota: Moose Mountain, an overly commercialized indoor mini-golf course at the Mall of America. I wanted to meet my new internet date in public in case, you know, he was an online serial killer. I even told Kristi, my younger sister by three years, who doubled as my roommate at the time, in a half joking, half serious tone to call the authorities if she didn't hear from me by 9:00 p.m. Luckily for me, Nick was not the "Twin Cities Torturer," but instead, my future husband.

Our affair of the heart was an easy one. When Nick's warm eyes first locked with mine, his brows raised in pleasant surprise, and a smile widened across his fair-skinned face, revealing his bright, white teeth that contrasted against his bright-blue collared shirt. I walked toward him against the backdrop of a food court filled with smells of Cinnabon and slushies and the muffled screams of riders of an indoor roller coaster, when I sensed that something about him was different and exciting. In our first glance, like in every good fairy tale, our adventure had begun.

While playing putt-putt, I asked Nick all the inappropriate questions, as I was known to do. No longer wanting to waste time kissing more frogs, I barraged him with inquiries.

"What are your thoughts on the welfare system?"

"I think it has its place."

Good. "Democrat or Republican?"

"I would call myself fiscally conservative and socially liberal."

Okay. "In your profile, you mentioned you were Christian; do you still go to church?"

"I'm a retired Lutheran."

My agnostic heart swooned.

Over a chain-food restaurant dinner of salmon and steak, we talked about books, his favorite, *Man's Search for Meaning,* while I professed, I couldn't pick just one. My love for stories was one reason why I wanted to become a therapist. Admittedly, I could have answered his question more honestly but held back because I was embarrassed to admit the book that had led me to meeting him.

For Christmas a few months before, my Aunt Mary had given me a copy of *Eat, Pray, Love,* Elizabeth Gilbert's memoir of travels to find herself. My forty-something aunt, always perceptive, noticed I had become melancholy over the past year. Within the span of a few weeks, I was fired five months into my first job out of college, dumped by a friend's ex-boyfriend I was wrongly sleeping with, and most devastatingly, my grandpa died. I fell into a deep depression.

My aunt, recovering from cancer with her prematurely wrinkled and worn, pale face framed by her once-black, now-growing-in gray hair, watched as I thumbed through the book as others opened Christmas gifts in a 1970s ranch-style living room. Aunt Mary leaned over my shoulder from behind with a glass of red wine in one hand and whispered in my ear, "I think you'll like it. It might give you some perspective."

And it did. I was inspired by Gilbert's candid struggles with life and the shadow of depression that can sometimes loom large over it. Her book gave me permission to allow myself a do-over for my previous lack of direction, and I enrolled in a graduate school therapy program to help myself and others address those demons that sometimes lurk inside.

Secretly though, another part of me wanted to be a writer and chronicle my own life in a similar way as Gilbert did, but as a twenty-five-year-old, soon-to-be masters-of-social-work student, I didn't have any real story to tell or the cash to travel the world to create one. I decided instead to start online dating, with the intent to write a book about all my crazy dates that would end, most likely, in noteworthy disasters. The title was to be *Lindsey's Month of Love*, but the book never came to be because my first date with Nick was the last online date I'd ever go on.

Looking back, I could say it was love at first sight, but at the time I was hesitant to believe it was true. Maybe I was afraid that if I did, I would jinx it. I think Nick was too, even though he didn't believe in things like luck or hexes. Years later, I asked him why he ended the date so early our first night, giving me a hug instead of going in for a kiss.

He replied, "Because I didn't want to ruin a good thing."

Nick and I might have been tentative at first, but everyone else in my circle knew he was my Prince Charming.

I've been told there's a shift that happens in the aura of a person when they meet their special someone. Even if you can't see auras, as I can't, you can still feel the movement in a person's energy when they fall in love. Maybe it's in the way their new lover's name leaves their lips, or in the micromovements on their face as you catch their smirk turn into a swoon.

My mother claimed it was the sound of my voice when I said Nick's name; my sister probably saw changes in my aura (she's into that stuff); friends noted how much more I smiled since starting to date him.

One late summer's evening, early in our relationship, while washing dishes after dinner in my apartment kitchen, I started humming the melody of *You Are My Sunshine* when Nick walked into the room. A warm flush crept across my cheeks as I faced him. I continued anyway, with a change to the lyrics. I sang to him in my off-key voice, "You are my boyfriend, my online boyfriend—" He rolled his eyes as I giggled through the rest and finished with, "Please don't take my online boyfriend away." My stare fixed on his as he moved closer, and I asked instead of singing, "You're not going to take my online boyfriend away, are you?"

Scooping his arms around my waist, he held my gaze and paused. Both of us wondered what the other was thinking. He pressed his lean muscular body against mine. Like puzzle pieces, I fit perfectly nuzzled into his neck. His minty breath was warm against the skin of my nape as he whispered in my ear, "Never." Pulling me tighter to him, he kissed my parted lips, softly, slowly, and longingly. It was then that I *felt* the shift in my own aura and knew what everyone else already saw. He was the one.

We did everything the "right" way. When a pseudo-perfectionist (me) and a rule follower (him) fall in love, life proceeds as planned. One year after our first date we whispered, "I love you." Check. Two years forward, we moved in together. Check. Three years went by, and we were engaged. Check. Four years passed, and we were married. Check. Everything worked out in order, just like the nursery rhyme I had sung as a child foreshadowed. "First comes love, then comes marriage . . ." Then, five years later we bought a house and on move-in day, I couldn't wait to share with him our newest adventure. "Then comes baby in a baby carriage."

I was pregnant.

chapter 2

A BABY IN
A BABY CARRIAGE

I had planned to tell Nick about the news of us expecting a baby once we got the keys to our new home. I envisioned handing him the positive pregnancy test in the spare room with pale-green walls that still smelled of fresh paint and had been set aside for our future child. But I couldn't wait because I was bursting with the secret news.

In the bathroom of our old home, then an empty, one-bedroom, downtown Minneapolis condo where we waited out the rain before we could move into our new four-bedroom one in the suburbs, I tied a small delicate green bow around the positive pregnancy test I had hidden in the pocket of my purse from the night before. Perfecting the bow, I tightened the ribbon and placed its edge eye level with the plus sign in the test window. Emerging from the bathroom with my hands behind my back, I slowly stepped toward Nick seated on the bare mattress in the middle of the empty floor. Standing above him, I silently placed it in his hands.

Nick glanced down, noticed the plus sign, and became wide-eyed. For a moment, he was still before he looked back at me.

"I'm going to be a dad?" He whispered his words through happy tears as he stood.

"Yes!" I nodded with a twinkling smile before we embraced.

Teary-eyed and innocent was how we started our journey into parenthood. Totally trusting of the universe and sure everything would go as planned because it had so far. What could go wrong? Our baby was a sure thing.

Learning I was pregnant didn't stop me from wondering if I'd made the right choice to become a mother. My gynecologist must have read my mind while looking at my vulva. With her eyes framed by my bent knees in stirrups, she looked up over the paper sheet laid across my stomach separating us as an emotional shield of sorts and without prompting said, "It's okay if you're still feeling hesitant about parenthood. Most new moms do."

Instead of feeling awkward about having this conversation while my doctor inspected my vagina, I fixated on the fact she had used the word *mom*. I didn't *feel* like one and recalled how I never desired to be one.

Growing up, I wasn't the girl who played with dolls or babysat. Kristi had rocked her Cabbage Patch Kids to sleep and dressed up in our mother's high heels. I, however, was more like Pippi Longstocking in spirit and looks—a rambunctious tomboy with red hair and freckles. I was the girl who refused to wear dresses or brush her hair, preferring a bumpy ponytail over perfected pigtails, and played basketball with the neighborhood boys on country gravel driveways instead of playing pretend house. I was not the type of girl interested in parenthood.

My mother didn't make wanting to become one any easier. Not because she was a villainous mother whose mistakes I did not want to repeat, but because she embodied motherhood. When I remember my mom from childhood, I always see her in the garden on hot, late summer afternoons with dirty knees and mud-stained hands as my sister and I, both school-age children, encircled her barefoot and wild as Mom dug in the damp, dewy earth, creating and nurturing life, urging it to grow. She hummed while she worked, hands deep in dirt, spreading fertilized soil made of the composted dinner scraps of carrot tops and potato peels. I watched in wonder as she helped Mother Earth facilitate the cycle of life in our own backyard.

The tune I like to think she sang in the sunlight with her hands tending to the soil was the same one I once altered for Nick. The lyrics lived in our house on the walls, spoken often in the words between my parents and in the handwritten letters my father left for her when he traveled for weeks at a time for work.

You knew when a note on the counter from Dad was for Mom because it would start with "My Sunshine," a pet name designated for her only. Except for at bedtime, in the years when we were young, Mom would share her endearment as she sat beside my bed, her curly, shoulder-length blond hair framing her blue eyes behind her '80s, coke-bottle glasses as she sang the song, "You Are My Sunshine" to me. And with a kiss on the forehead, she would whisper *sweet dreams*—all so naturally and so sure in her role as a mother, as *my* mother.

Even before she was a mother, she was certain in her desire to become one. After two years of trying unsuccessfully to conceive a child, my dad confided in my mom that he didn't need to have children. My mother's reply was one so sure in her natural inclination toward maternity: "I wouldn't feel complete if we didn't."

It was a sentiment I hadn't agreed with and still didn't quite understand. Maybe her conviction for motherhood sturdily grew from a place of longing, from losing her own mother when she was sixteen to a sudden and deadly brain aneurysm? Wherever her certainty came from, I did not inherit it.

As a child, I saw my mother's role and found it limiting and bland. It was my father, the once fighter pilot turned international aviator, who I wanted to become. I had no desire to fly F-16 and A-10 planes as he did, but I yearned for a life like his. I wanted to see the world and go on daring adventures like in *Peter Pan*, the opposite of my mom, who was more like Laura Ingalls Wilder in *Little House on the Prairie*.

Dad would come home from long trips away to places like Germany, Kuwait, or the Panama Canal, and Kristi and I would run to the front door to greet him. Still wearing his pea-green flight suit, he gave us tight hugs and warm kisses, then everyone would head up the stairs behind him as he carried a flight helmet in one hand and a large green duffle bag full of treasures in the other.

Over the years, wooden Russian nesting dolls and their clones, along with porcelain figurines dressed in colorful polleras lined the shelves in my bedroom. Cocoa-scented German chocolates not available in the States were also pulled from his satchel. My favorite gift—a fluffy, Steiff stuffed panda bear made in Germany—lived many years between my arms at night. I had recently found it stored in my parents' basement and set it aside to give to the baby growing in my belly.

It's as if I was raised by Mother Earth and Father Sky. My mother was grounded in all things earthbound. My father was called to "stir the star-filled cauldrons of the sky, dance with moonbeams, and godlike, make the sun rise and set," as his own father, my grandfather, a radar observer after World War II and poet wrote of their shared love affair with the world above the horizon.

While my father chased sunsets and lived amongst moonbeams, my mother was left behind to tend to the garden of our family, to make sure my sister and I grew. I saw her as a caged bird, unable to fly, her wings clipped by children. But my mother did not feel caged, for she was secure in her nest. To me, it seemed motherhood was the end of the freedom to fly to the next adventure . . . until I met Nick and realized having children might be an adventure I would want to take with him. The thought of our separate DNA pieces combined into one little person became alluring. After years of disregarding motherhood, I embarked on it but with uncertainty.

At three months pregnant, I hadn't told my clients and coworkers yet. I covered my tiny bump with a large blouse as I sat in my small square office in my swivel therapist chair across from my client, Jessica, who was just a few years older than me and in her midthirties. Sober for two years, she had recently married. Jessica took a seat on the cream-colored couch, placed her Coach purse next to a throw pillow, and crossed her knee-high boots, one over the other.

"I'm pregnant!" she exclaimed. She had just found out that morning and couldn't contain the news.

Smiling wide at her excitement, I congratulated her and asked all the obligatory questions before finishing with, "How do you feel?"

Brushing her curly, brunette hair off her shoulder, her matching brown eyes found my gaze. "Scared."

"Why?" I asked.

Her reply surprised me, "I'm a mom. My life has changed forever. It's like a light switch was turned on and no matter what happens, it can never be turned off again. From this point forward, I'm a parent. There is no taking that back."

I placed a hand on my concealed but stretched stomach, letting her realization settle inside me and start to become mine.

chapter 3

LOVE AT
FIRST SIGHT

Twenty weeks after move-in day, we watched as a pregnancy test plus sign had evolved into an outline of a baby that bounced around on an ultrasound screen above our heads in an exam room. I had been feeling flutters in my belly since about sixteen weeks, which was a welcomed reward for the previous fourteen of undergoing the misnomer of morning sickness and unrelenting fatigue. Even though I could no longer button my pants, the concept of having a baby under them didn't really sink in until that moment when we saw a small human on the monitor doing gymnastics that matched the movement I felt inside. And as the old worn-out rocking horse said to the Velveteen Rabbit, now that our baby was real, they could never become unreal again, for real "lasts for always."

"Your baby looks perfect," our sonographer said at the end of the forty-five-minute anatomy scan. From behind my shoulder, Nick let out a sigh of relief.

"Would you like to know the sex of the baby?" she asked, while continuing to move the cool, blue gel-covered magic wand over my bare belly like a fortune teller waving her hands over a crystal ball. We replied in unison with a simple nod as we intently watched for shapes of genitals in the black-and-white blur of a tiny person swimming in suspended space on the screen. The sonographer then pointed to the "hamburger" proof of three white lines on the monitor that our baby had female anatomy.

"It's a girl!" she confirmed with a smile.

"A girl?" I replied as I felt *her* flutter, instantly falling prey to the dream that the sex of a baby brings to a parent's imagination.

Turning toward Nick, I watched his cheeks flush. The flood of emotions over the realization he had a daughter was slowly sinking in, the weight was written upon his wide-eyed and tear-filled face as he envisioned what his future life would hold. Baby years of three a.m. awakenings with him rocking her to sleep that would in no time turn into adolescent years of late-night worries wondering where she was after curfew. I imagined our futures with her simultaneously. Thinking about how sweet it would be for me to peek in on daddy and daughter tea parties for two, to one day witnessing him get teary eyed in the same way he was in front of the ultrasound screen, when we waved goodbye after dropping her off at college.

"We're having a girl!" he finally said.

With wet eyes I replied softly, "Yeah."

After wiping the gel off my belly, the technician turned on the lights and handed me a flimsy envelope with shiny black-and-white pictures inside. The first photos of our baby girl.

"Congratulations. *She* looks perfect!" the sonographer said again as we left the room.

Nick pushed the button for the elevator in the lobby while I inspected the pictures of our baby. With his hands in his pockets, Nick watched me imprint every inch of her profile to memory, "Well it's official then. *She* is Nora," he proclaimed.

We had tried to agree on a baby's name a few weeks before. After hours of early pregnancy spent looking through woody-smelling hand-me-down baby books and online searches, we had easily chosen a name for a boy. Deciding on a girl's name proved to be more difficult. We made a list in a spiral notebook with ten to fifteen different options scribbled inside, some in his handwriting, some in mine. None of them seemed to do.

Then the night before the anatomy scan, while Nick slept next to me in bed, my mother's middle name, Norine, came to mind. I quickly patted my nightstand to find my phone. In the darkness, I typed in the six letters to Google—Norine. "A woman of honor" glowed from my screen. It was an older name, not in fashion now, which made it more appealing. It was Irish in origin, just like Nick and I were, to some degree. My initial thought was Norine was too formal, but after more scrolling, I found a shorter version—Nora. Nora meant both honor and light. We could name her Norine and call her Nora for short. I couldn't wait until morning to ask Nick his thoughts on the name, so I reached over and gave him a little nudge to wake him. "What about Nora?"

In the stillness of nearing midnight, I heard him shuffle under the sheets before he paused as if he was still asleep. But with his back facing me he broke the dark silence. "Yeah, I like it."

Nora she was to be.

But next to the large fake fern in the monochromatic clinic lobby I was scared to make it official. "Are you sure we want to use her name so soon?"

"Why not? That's the name we chose for a girl." Nick had a look of confusion brewing on his brow, wanting an explanation for my sudden hesitation.

I didn't tell him that after we agreed upon what to call her for the rest of her life, I went to sleep envisioning her whole future as Nora. I saw those letters on her birth certificate, birthday cards, report cards, and wedding invites. I also didn't tell him I saw her name on a gravestone. Not in a negative way but in a dignified way of a life well lived. But now, as we considered making it official, the memory of the vision of the name *Nora* on a headstone gave me goosebumps. All I could think of as we waited for the elevator, looking at our baby's first photo was, what if she doesn't get to use it?

Not knowing how to explain the jumbled thoughts and feelings floating through my mind, I simply acquiesced. From the moment he pressed the elevator button for the ground floor and the doors closed, she was officially Nora. After all, we already loved her, and a baby needed a name.

Falling in love with Nora was like falling in love with each other all over again. It happened almost subconsciously, like breathing.

"Do you want to feel her move?" I asked Nick, a week after our anatomy scan as I sat sweating in an oversized sofa chair. We were visiting my parents at my childhood home in rural Wisconsin on a sweltering August afternoon. I was mindful not to use Nora's name in front of my mom, sitting adjacent to me on the loveseat, folding down the corners of a gardening magazine. We wanted to keep Nora's name a secret until she arrived.

"Sure." Nick got up from lying on the carpeted floor where he had been reading the news on his iPhone of Mitt Romney choosing his running mate for the upcoming presidential election. Walking toward me, he bent a knee to be by my side. "Do you think I'll be able to feel her this time?"

Nick hadn't yet felt Nora's movements. They seemed so strong and distinctive to me, but they were difficult to detect from the outside. For a few weeks, Nora and I had developed our own game of poke and push. I would prod at her with my fingers pressed firmly against my belly, and she would respond back with a kick or a jab. The ebb and flow of our push and poke sessions were like the tide. I was the moon and she, the waves, responding to each other's calls for connection from across the veil of space and time.

With the added weight of pregnancy pushing me heavier into the cushy chair, I was hoping Nick would finally be able to partake in our game. I rolled my cotton tank top up so he could place his hand on my bare belly in the spot where she had just wiggled. His hand was warm against my skin as he waited for her to kick back against his palm.

"Did you feel that?" I tensed with excitement.

Nick shook his head with a disappointed frown. Still feeling a continuous jab of what I assumed must have been a foot or a knee, I moved his hand from my belly button toward the left side of my midsection and pushed his fingers into my skin. "Try here," I insisted.

Then, there was a *pop* from within, and Nick's face glowed with a grin that stretched from ear to ear. His twinkling eyes turned toward mine. "Is that her?"

I smiled wide in return, noticing from the corner of my eye my mom touching away a tear before I nodded toward Nick. He was finally able to participate in our now three-player game. Lingering longer in the spot where he had first felt her move, he leaned in to talk to her for the first time.

"Hi, baby girl. It's your daddy."

Her wiggles and squirms increased in strength over the next twenty weeks of pregnancy. As my belly grew, so did our excitement. With each poke, we could feel her coming from her internal world into ours. Summer quickly turned into fall, where our country, too, was committing to the motto of moving forward by reelecting Barack Obama for a second term. We hunkered down the rest of autumn; the leaves fell until the branches were bare, and the frigid winds of winter brought us closer to Nora's due date, only a day away. We inched closer to the moment when our eyes would lock with hers, and we would fall in love with Nora all over again, but this time at first sight.

The late afternoon of Christmas Day had turned to dusk. The neighbor's holiday lights twinkled brightly outside our bedroom window in winter's snowy darkness. Nick had his cheek on my belly as he continued talking to Nora, just as he did the first time twenty weeks before.

"Our bags are packed, and your room is ready. You can come anytime now!"

In reply, Nora kicked him through the wall of my skin.

We both laughed, and Nick said, "I'll take that as a 'Not yet, Dad.'"

Resuming his reading, Nick snuggled next to me under the warm comforter as I continued spending time with Nora, playing our game of poke and push. Her movements reassured me she was there. But even with her consistent commotion coming from within, I couldn't shake the feeling that something wasn't right. Noticing the skin on my belly rise and fall as she rolled, I asked, "What if something goes wrong?"

"Everything will be fine," Nick replied firmly, closing his book. His voice was gentle, but I could sense frustration. Nick never liked my anxiety, and I had a lot of it. My incessant nervousness to him was a sign of insecurity. It also made him feel helpless, as he didn't know how to fix my concerns.

"Why do you always have to worry so much?"

"How do you know it will be okay?" I snapped, without adding, *Because something seems not right.*

There was this *feeling* that gnawed at me, like the feeling you get when the phone rings and you know before you answer that the person on the other end is going to deliver bad news.

Something had shifted, was different inside, like how it *felt* in the moments before I peed on a pregnancy test. Almost like a magic trick, something that once wasn't there suddenly was, and the pregnancy test confirmed it. Maybe nine months ago, it was the slight nauseousness hovering in the back of my throat, or how I would get winded after climbing a single flight of stairs at work. But underneath those physical symptoms, an intuition told me something was there that wasn't before—something had drifted into my being. I just *knew* I was pregnant before the plus sign appeared, like my family and friends just *knew* Nick was the one for me. Fast forward to being almost forty weeks pregnant and overdue, I *knew* it—*felt* it in my bones—that the something settled inside of me seemed as though it was drifting away, like a feather upon a breeze.

"Everything will be okay," he said again. "It's normal to be nervous right now. I know you're worried because tomorrow is your due date and nothing has happened yet, but that doesn't mean anything bad will happen." Nick tried calming my fears. His steady nature was one of the reasons I married him as it balanced out my own neurosis. "Everything will be all right."

But my apprehension remained. It came from such an innate place I couldn't find the words to explain it. I *felt* something wasn't right or was about not to be. I wanted to tell Nick about my déjà vu experience on my thirtieth birthday two weeks before. While walking around the block with Georgie before the first snowfall, a vision swept over me with certainty that I would be pregnant three times. I wasn't afraid of this calm knowing, but I didn't understand it. I was thirty-eight weeks pregnant with Nora at the time, and Nick and I never wanted more than two children. I couldn't comprehend why I would be pregnant twice more after this. I kept the memory to myself and chalked it up to an anxious mind, as Nick would have if I had told him.

Instead, I murmured, "Okay." I hoped agreeing with him would trick myself into believing him. Feeling Nora move again, I couldn't shake the *sense* that something was about to go terribly wrong.

Nick could tell I was not completely satisfied with his answer and with newfound empathy, took me into his arms. Letting myself lean into his chest, I soaked in his musky-pine scent as he tightened his squeeze and repeated in a gentler tone, "Everything is good right now. We're happy."

And I felt Nora move one more time.

chapter 4

THE LAST TIME

Thick snow crunched beneath my swollen feet. My breath was heavy and quick as we trekked through the woods down by the frozen river. Two days past my due date, I was forty-plus weeks pregnant and forty pounds heavier. The extra baby weight I carried had become too much for my average frame to hold. Not able to let go of any poundage, I instead lightened my load by shedding the weight of my worries. Nick's reassurance from a few days before had been enough to quell my concerns. Instead of worrying about the future, I shifted my anxious energy into working toward being in the future, by trying to bring about labor, to no avail.

In the last week, I had eaten pieces of pineapple, my least favorite fruit, engaged in awkward full-term pregnancy sex, and spent an afternoon climbing flights of stairs at the office in between therapy sessions, hoping it would cause a contraction or two. But nothing worked. Nora seemed content to live her life inside my womb.

Fluffy snowflakes laid against barren birch tree branches we hiked under. Chunks of ice occasionally fell to the forest floor, succumbing to the added weight of winter. Every step I took was getting harder to take with an infant inside me. Having trouble maintaining pace with Nick, who was slightly ahead, I exhaled heavily. My breath became thick mist that hung in the air.

Nora moved between my breathy steps; she always did—her full-grown body of newborn size twisting and sliding against mine. Stopping suddenly, I leaned forward as I inhaled through the pain of Braxton Hicks' contractions that her somersaults induced, cradling my belly in response. I hugged both hands around my pelvis as if she might fall out during each muscle tightening. My arms moved instinctively to the position of protecting her.

Nick, noticing I was no longer by his side, had stopped up ahead and came back. "Are you okay?"

"Yes," I huffed, while hunched over, still clasping my belly as I worked to slow my breathing.

"Do you want to turn around?"

Feeling the small practice contraction subside, I stood up. "Let's keep going. It's nice out. It will probably be our last hike before she comes." I started trekking down the trail again, keeping one hand cupped under my caterpillar in her cocoon.

Nick held my other hand. Sensing something was missing under my mitten, he asked, "Where is your new ring?"

He had gotten me a right-handed ring for my thirtieth birthday. When I picked it out at the jewelry counter, Nick told me the gift was a symbol of bringing our child into this world and referred to it as my "mother ring."

"My fingers are too swollen to wear it. It's in the box in my dresser at home."

"*Hmm*," he replied, his eyes focused down the trail watching George, who was off his leash bouncing in and out of the snow-covered soil, sniffing for scents winter had buried. "You should pack it in the hospital bag for after her birth."

I nodded, loving his suggestion. Nick seemed so secure in his decision to become a father, never once questioning if we should have gone down the path of parenthood like I did.

It was Nick, not I, who exuded excitement about becoming a

parent. He read all the baby books and parenting books, too. He highlighted passages with yellow markers and shared with me the ways in which we were going to parent Nora from age six months to sixteen years old. He researched cribs and car seats and sent in all the recall notification cards as we purchased the items we needed. Nick strapped an old teddy bear of mine into the car seat and took it to the police station to make sure it was safely installed in our newly purchased, practical, four-door crossover. He had proudly traded in the not-so-practical, two-door, sports car he used to own. His transition into parenthood came naturally to him. Trusting the processes of becoming a parent like a caterpillar must trust their chrysalis to become a butterfly. While I constantly contemplated my uncertainty about becoming a mom, he was ready to be a dad.

The tags of George's collar clinked together like jingle bells, echoing through the frozen forest as we continued down the trail. Feeling Nora push against my belly button, I pondered, "Do you think she will come before our induction date?" It was set for that Tuesday, the first of the year.

"A New Year's Baby!" our doctor exclaimed earlier that morning at our appointment. She then stripped my membranes in hopes of bringing about labor, causing my mucus plug to fall out, but it resulted in yet another failed attempt at nudging things along.

"I hope so! I would love to get the tax credit for this year." Nick and I both chuckled at his usual fixation on all things fiscal.

Switching to a more somber tone, I shared, "I want her to come before the induction date. I always envisioned waking up in the middle of the night and rushing to the hospital." Looking down at my winter boots sinking in the deep snow, I continued, "I'm kind of disappointed it won't happen that way." My swollen feet rubbed against the seams, which just added to my annoyance of being overdue. January first, Tuesday of next week, seemed like ages away from that Friday afternoon.

"We still have a few days. It could happen." Nick was forever the optimist, which paired well with my inherent pessimism.

We walked through the snow in silence a little longer before I confessed, "I'm tired."

"Do you want to head back?"

"That's not what I meant." I took a deep breath of cold air that exhaled as a weighted sigh. "I'm tired of being pregnant. It's so hard. And I hate the changes that are happening to my body. I feel like pregnancy is an extreme version of puberty all over again." I didn't tell Nick I had researched the psychological term for the transformation from maiden to mother—*matrescence*, the physical, psychological, and emotional changes a woman goes through to become a mother. It sounded a lot like adolescence and was probably filled with more hormones. "It's awkward and uncomfortable and happens so fast." I sounded like Alice in Wonderland, trying to explain unsuccessfully to the caterpillar why being so many different sizes in a day is rather confusing, except for me it had been 283 days of changing my form. "I just want her to be here."

"Me, too." Nick squeezed my hand as we switched directions, working our way back up the trail toward the parking lot.

Over recent dinners with friends, Nick had often said, "We are ready to become parents." It was his acknowledgment that at thirty-five, five years my senior, he was secretly afraid he was getting too old to start parenthood. We had waited until the "responsible" time in our life to have children. And just like the rule followers and planners we respectively were, we also had everything prepared for Nora's arrival. The premade meals were in the deep freeze, the nursery decorated with the crib assembled, and baby clothes sorted into dresser drawers stacked next to fresh diapers, all eagerly waiting to be used. The nest was ready, my husband was ready, and I was more than ready for pregnancy to be over, but I was seated on a fence about motherhood, questioning what I was about to become.

Curious about his response to my concerns, and in need of some reassurance, I again unloaded my worries about our chosen future onto him. "Do you think we made the right choice?"

"Right choice?" He stopped abruptly in the snow. His vision narrowed, "About what? The induction?"

"No, not that," I said, hoping my soft tone would take away some of the tension I saw tightening between his temples. "Do you ever worry about . . .?" Taking a minute to collect my thoughts, I looked away, trying to find the words to continue carefully, not to further frustrate him. "How having a baby is going to change us?"

He forcefully exhaled the crisp air with his response, "This is what we wanted . . . to have a family."

"Yes," I said, nodding my head toward the path and not him. "It is."

"Are you sure? It's a little too late to start second guessing." His brow furrowed as he questioned my questions.

"Yes," I said again, not confidently, but firmly enough for Nick to be satisfied with my answer, letting the conversation quell into silence. But I was not persuaded by my own reply. With motherhood on the horizon, just past the next sunset or two, I still wondered if being a mother was for me. It seemed a little late to second guess things, but maybe all mothers on the precipice of metamorphosis felt this way. Maybe it was part of becoming a mother.

Changing the subject Nick stated, "George is almost back to the car. I better catch him before he gets to the parking lot. I'll meet you up there?"

I nodded, and he hurried ahead. Moving slowly along the trail behind him, I found it hard to breathe as I slogged through the snow. Small flakes started to fall faintly from the sky. I stopped unexpectedly for no apparent reason and turned to face the woods behind me. The snowflakes were momentarily mesmerizing, like the soft, slow, gentle snowflakes reserved for snow globes and quaint Christmas movie endings, where everything seemed too good to be true.

The warmth of the afternoon winter sun retreated as it dipped below the horizon. Snowflakes kissed my face, causing me to shiver. Something—a voice or feeling—told me to linger a little longer in this liminal space on the precipice of parenthood, even though my feet tingled with numbness, and Nora's weight pulled at my spine. "Remember this," the voice said, "this is the last time things will be this way."

Suddenly, Nora kicked with her usual reassuring force, and with it, my desire for motherhood bloomed boldly from within. Motherhood settled within my soul. Cupping my hands under my round middle, I hugged her once more from the outside in. "Hi, sweet girl," I softly said in response. Then, right on cue, like she always did, Nora kicked back, one last time.

The next day, Nora had still not arrived. That evening, after watching a movie in front of a warm, crackling fire, Nick and I retired to bed early. It was only eight p.m., but I was drained and exhausted, having felt "off" ever since I woke from the nap I had taken earlier in the afternoon. I sensed labor was soon approaching, but did not yet share my inkling with Nick, as I did not want to get his hopes up or mine.

As we ascended the stairs, I stopped just like I did in the woods the day before, but this time it was my own voice I heard that blurted out, "I'm not ready for this!" My momentary contentment with impending parenting had floated away, like a butterfly on a breeze.

Nick laughed and said playfully this time, "You better be. There is a newborn in your belly."

Once again, I was aware of this liminal space we lingered in . . . this strange place of crossing over and leaving something behind but not yet fully in our new form. In all seriousness, I replied, "This will be the last time it's like this."

Nick scoffed as I continued, seeming to find humor in my last-minute alarm.

"There won't be any more nights where it's just you and me. No more holidays just the two of us. It makes me sad. Isn't it for you?"

"No," he said gently. "I'm ready for us to expand our family and our love. Now, let's go to bed." He waved his hand, gesturing for me to follow him up the stairs.

And that's when I realized I was scared. But of what? I wasn't sure. Something seemed to have changed over the last day. Instead of preparing to add something to our family, I sensed something was dying. Maybe my youth? *Change is hard for everyone. Starting something new is always the death of something old*, I told myself to quiet my nerves. It didn't work. My body wasn't convinced to calm itself as it *knew* something was already different or was about to be. I *felt* it in my bones.

I couldn't sleep. Nick was out the moment his head hit the pillow. *Waiting can be so exhausting,* I thought as I watched him snore. But I struggled to get comfortable in bed. My large belly caused my back to hurt more than usual. I tossed and turned for over an hour and began wondering when I last noticed Nora move. I had been so tired and achy, I hadn't paid attention to her that day. Placing my hand on my belly she slept in, I tried recalling the last time she told me she was there.

Thinking through the events of that evening a tightness rose in my throat. *Did I feel her move during dinner?* She always danced around after a meal. *What about while watching a movie on the couch?* I couldn't recall. All I could remember was the coolness of the ice pack against my spine, easing my back spasms. *When was the last time she kicked?* Flipping and flopping from left to right, I laid my hand again on the opposite side of my stomach while replaying the day, desperate for her to move. My rustling must have woken George. His collar jingled as he circled around in bed to reposition himself. The sound of his clinking collar reminded me Nora was very active during our hike the afternoon before. I let out a long exhale of relief. She was moving yesterday; she must be all right. What could happen in a day's time? My previously constricted muscles began relaxing, and I sank into the sheets.

Babies slow down toward birth. I remembered this inaccurate and deadly myth well-meaning doctors and moms on internet message boards often said about the final days of pregnancy. I tried convincing myself this was why I had not noticed her as much that day.

Just for added reassurance, I changed positions again in bed, hoping that my motions would wake her. Laying on my right side with my left hand hugging her from the outside, I pressed my sweaty fingers into the soft part of my large belly to get Nora's attention, waiting anxiously for her to respond.

Ten minutes went by without a jab, kick, or even a squirm. I tried poking at her again. This time more forcefully, as it was odd for her to not return my prods. *She's being stubborn*, I thought, *after all, she is my daughter.* But this wasn't like her. Nora was never quiet for more than forty-five-minute stretches. The tightness in my throat returned along with the stiffness in my shoulders. My concern at her lack of response intensified. Deciding to get up and move around, thinking it might help the situation, I went downstairs in search of a snack to wake her.

Walking down the steps that led to the kitchen, I didn't need to flick on the light switch as the moonlight let itself in through the windows and flooded the walls of each room. Opening the refrigerator, I found a piece of fudge alone on a back shelf under an eerie fluorescent glow, leftover from the holiday celebrations a few days before. Unwrapping it from the plastic, I ate it quickly. Then to wash the stuck sugar from my teeth, I moved to the kitchen sink and poured myself a glass of ice-cold water. Nora was still silent inside.

Downing my drink, I glanced out the window above the faucet where my gaze was pulled out onto the front lawn toward the tree with the small bird feeder illuminated by the remnants of the day-old full moon reflecting off the newly fallen snow below. The moon in her fullness was calling to me, reminding me of the feminine phases she morphed through during the month—first maiden, then mother, and finally fading into a crone. There was either a blessing or a curse in her moonlight cutting through the darkness.

Shivers shimmied down my spine at the sight of her fullness beginning to wane. A clue lingered in Mother Moon's burning brightness that I couldn't decode. Something was similar between us. I assumed it was being on the cusp of transitioning into something entirely new, from maiden to mother. But if that was her message, then why did I feel cautious about the crone she was becoming? Squinting, I focused on the small sliver of her that had dipped into darkness.

Standing in the moon's glow that flooded the front of the window, I laid my hands on my stomach as I waited for Nora to kick like she always did after a sweet treat. Anxiously anticipating her movement, I took in the beauty of the moonlight reflecting off the mountains of snow lining our sidewalk when suddenly, there was a soft wiggle, and another small sway inside me. I let out a deep sigh, and my muscles loosened in relief.

"Thank you," I said out loud to Nora, without breaking my gaze with Mother Moon.

Just then, the walls of my belly hardened as pain circled back to compress against my spine. Grasping the kitchen counter, I braced myself through the constriction. It wouldn't be long now. My contractions were coming, and so was she.

Making my way slowly back up the stairs I crawled into bed next to Nick who was still snoring. Taking the advice from our birthing class coach to get some rest at home while in the early stages of labor, I tried settling in for some sleep. With my head on the pillow, I focused on counting her kicks. Placing a hand once more on my belly, and in the position I had started in over an hour before, I tallied her dim movements, one, a drawn-out pause, and then two. It was taking longer than usual to get to ten, but by the third weak motion I was satisfied enough to fall asleep. *Babies slow down when they get close to birth*, I regretfully reassured myself. Then she moved softly again within me, a fourth time. The last time.

chapter 5

I'M SORRY, THERE'S
NO HEARTBEAT

I woke to a scream from outside the bedroom window. Paralyzed by fear in bed, I waited for another, but none came. Nick did not hear it, as he was still soundly asleep. Cautiously, I went to the window and pulled back the heavy curtains—nothing except moonlight flooding the cold room like an unwanted guest. Its bright eerie beauty seemed intrusive, making me uneasy and restless. Quivers swept over my skin as I questioned if the noise was even real. Letting the curtain fall back into place, I shook my head as if trying to shake away a ghost.

What time is it? It had to be past midnight. I shuffled around the edges of the bed, searching for my phone on the nightstand. Its bold white numbers informed me it was a few minutes before two a.m. Fully awake, I noticed my bladder pushing on my pelvic floor. I headed toward the bathroom when a radiating pain washed down my hips toward the center of my back where the two tides of a throb met along my spine. This contraction was more intense than the one in the kitchen just a few hours earlier. Walking through the ache, I reached the toilet where I hoped peeing would relieve the built-up pressure, but the pain continued.

Hunched over, I waddled back into bed beside Nick, who I wasn't yet ready to wake. Sitting propped up against pillows, I tried breathing through the pulsating tightness that spread throughout my lower body, making it difficult to move. Realizing then that it was time to contact the hospital, I dialed their number.

"I think I'm in labor," I whispered into the phone after the nurse with a nasally voice answered.

"How far along are you?" she asked, after I recited my name and date of birth.

I could hear her typing as I replied, "I'm four days past my due date."

"Is the baby moving?" My muscles clenched at her question, as if bracing for the blow of an oncoming car before a crash, but I wasn't sure why.

"No." I paused and instinctively put my free hand on my belly with concern. "But I just woke up."

"When was the last time you felt the baby move?" she repeated.

My eyebrows perked up with unexpected enthusiasm when I remembered Nora's muted movements before I fell asleep. "Right before I went to bed. Around nine."

"Good," she said, as I heard her continuing to hit the keys on her computer through the phone. "How far apart are the contractions, and on a scale of one to ten, how would you rate the pain?"

"I'm not sure how far apart the contractions are. I think I've been having them since early evening, but the pain is more intense. I would rate it as . . . umm . . . a six, I guess?"

"Okay, well it sounds like it's time to come in," she conveyed with a chirpiness as she informed me of her final assessment. "We'll be waiting for you!"

Hanging up the phone, I gently nudged Nick's shoulders. With his eyes still closed he asked, "What did they say?" His alertness startled me, realizing he had heard the whole conversation.

"She said it's time to come in."

Turning to face me, he smiled through drowsy eyes. I did not mind his stale breath as he croaked, "We're going to have a baby!"

We took our time getting ready to leave because the nurse said not to rush. Slowly, I inserted each of my legs into a pant hole as I struggled to get dressed. The constant pressure on my tailbone made it difficult with Nora's spine feeling as if it was grinding, like teeth, against mine.

Nick dressed quickly, wetted down his cowlicked hair, and grabbed the hospital bag before going outside to warm up the car while I finished brushing my teeth. Putting the toothbrush away, the taste of mint lingered in my mouth as I closed the medicine cabinet door. I took one last look at my profile in the bathroom mirror and ran my hands over my watermelon-sized midsection that hung heavily out from underneath my maternity shirt, where Nora waited inside. I would leave this house tonight as one person and return an entirely different one. A family of two was about to become a family of three.

"Are you ready?" Nick yelled from downstairs.

"Yeah!" I replied, as I stroked my belly, soaking in my round reflection, and looking back at me one last time. I was ready . . . not only to leave to have a baby, but to become a mother. Something had shifted in the hours I had slept. The hesitation had evaporated, and excitement had settled in where apprehension once lived.

"I'll be right there," I replied, making my way down the hall where I passed Nora's nursery.

Stepping inside the little green room, I stole a moment there before we left to imagine all that awaited it. I could see so clearly our future nights. Nora would wake for feedings in her crib under the paper crane mobile that hung above her bed, fluttering softly in the silver moonlight. I would comfort her by singing her back to sleep in the rocking chair where my mother had comforted me in the same way. I recited Margaret Wise Brown's children's book *Goodnight Moon*. "Goodnight room, Goodnight moon," I said. "She'll be here soon," I whispered to the expectant nursery before shutting the door, hearing the soft latch of the doorknob, as if she was already sleeping inside.

"All set?" Nick asked, with his hand on the handle of the door to the garage. Adorned in his bulky, warm, winter gear, he looked like he was going on a snowmobiling trip rather than to the hospital.

"Yup. I can't believe we're going to do this. We're really going to have a baby!"

"Yes!" he nodded with a grin, "Now let's go."

There were two ways to get to the hospital: take a right and go on the back roads, or go left, like Nick did, and take the highway. The car's engine hummed as its tires rotated over the road. The smell of exhaust mingled with the scent of musty dust coming from the car's heater. We were both quiet as Nick drove, not sure what to say to each other as we weren't sure what lay ahead.

Another contraction came that gripped my back as a wave of pain rose again over my mountainous midsection. The soft, morose, before-dawn melody coming from the stereo became too loud for my ears. "Can you turn the music off?" I asked, my hand clutching the passenger side door as my stomach constricted.

Nick obliged and reached for the radio, "You okay?"

"Yeah. I'll be okay." The contraction receded, but the pressure was painfully present. "Where is the bag?" I asked, struggling to look in the back seat, unable to contort myself far enough around to find it. Suddenly, I had become fretful that we overlooked something, and everything would go wrong.

"Relax, it's next to the car seat."

Straining, I tilted my head a little more backward and to the left, finally able to see it. The bag was hidden on the other side of the polka-dot, pink-and-gray car seat that would have Nora snuggled inside the next time we got in the car to drive home from the hospital. I smiled as I imagined our future so near, I could almost touch it.

Nick drove to the hospital entrance and dropped me off before he parked the car. I hadn't made it very far into the building when he caught up with me just past the second set of sliding glass doors. Together, we walked slowly to the maternity ward. Each step I took gradually intensified the cramps, like a vice opening my pelvic floor.

"Hi, I'm Lindsey Henke. I called about an hour ago. I'm in labor," I said, once reaching the nurse's station.

"Oh, good. Come on in," replied the woman, whose voice inflection matched the one from the phone. "We're ready for you. Let's get you set up in a room."

We followed the middle-aged nurse with the nasally voice into the delivery room that smelled like bitter undertones of bleach and clean cotton sheets when we entered. Politely, she handed me a polyester gown and smiled, "Put this on. Your labor nurse should be in shortly."

Changing out of my maternity clothes and into the blue-and-white small, checkered gown, I modeled my new attire for Nick. "I look like I'm wearing a tent," I told him as he tightened ties together behind my back. Both of us laughed at the awkwardness of my new outfit.

"You won't look like that much longer," Nick said, smiling wide with excitement before he kissed my cheek.

"Thank goodness," I replied, as I not-so-gracefully plopped onto the bed with starched white, folded-down sheets. "I just want her to be here."

A young, thirty-something nurse with long, straight, sandy hair interrupted our giggling as she entered the room. Wearing blue scrubs and a kind smile with caring green eyes, she introduced herself, before explaining the next steps of the labor process. "Let's get you set up." She patted the mattress with her palm. "Can you scooch up a little on the bed, please?"

Jostling my bottom back against the nook in the bed, the nurse maneuvered straps attached to monitors behind my torso and around my basketball-sized midsection to prepare me for labor. "Is this your first?" she asked, passing the time with niceties as she placed the familiar cool blue gel on the skin of my stomach.

Exchanging a proud glance with Nick, we responded in unison, "Yes."

"How exciting! Do you know the baby's sex?" Putting the bottle down on the table next to her, she placed the round fetal monitor on top of my bulging belly.

"It's a girl," I answered.

"How nice." She grinned as she searched around my stretched stomach with the disc to find Nora's pulse.

"Do you have children?" I asked in polite reply, as she repositioned the monitor.

But she did not respond. Suddenly silent, the nurse's smile had slipped away. Furrowing her eyebrows with intense focus, she fiddled with the volume on the speaker, attempting to hear a heartbeat that wasn't mine. Taking longer than I remembered it had at previous appointments, a wave of heat flushed my face a blotchy pink. I hesitantly asked, "Is everything okay?"

The nurse, now stone-faced, forced a smile. "Sometimes the heartbeat is hard to find."

My stomach dropped as she touched my hand and gave it a friendly, yet foreboding squeeze. "I'll be right back with the doctor, and we'll figure things out." Standing up from where she sat on the corner of the bed, she left a little too quickly for my liking.

Nervous, I reached toward Nick, seated in the chair next to

me, for comfort. "I'm scared. It normally doesn't take this long to find her heartbeat."

"Everything will be okay." He took my trembling hand in his. *Everything must be okay. We did everything right. I just worry too much.*

My body settled into a silent sway. I searched for the clock on the wall for reassurance. The little hand pointed toward three. It had been six hours since I had counted her muted movements before I fell asleep. With that memory, I gulped for air, but it felt like my lungs were filling with water. I had been asleep most of that time . . . that's why I hadn't noticed her move. *Everything is fine,* I repeated in my mind while my body continued sinking into the deep darkness of an unfamiliar ocean. *The doctor will know what to do.*

Less than three minutes later, our nurse returned to the room ahead of the obstetrician, rolling in a portable ultrasound machine behind her, looking somehow different than she did when she left. She flashed a stiff smile when she noticed I watched her every move, like a worried passenger watching a flight attendant for cues of an impending plane crash. Walking from the side of the room to the front of the bed, the nurse set up the ultrasound machine, unable to camouflage her concern.

"This is Dr.——" I tried focusing on the words she spoke, but it was hard to hear her over the pounding of my pulse. "He's going to take a look."

Through a fog, I nodded my head in response, though I swear my body froze. Nick moved from the chair to the side of my bed where we sat hip to hip. Feeling him place his hand on my shoulder, I bit my lip as I tried controlling the trembling tears that roared to be released.

The doctor with a mop of hair that fell over his thick glasses wore green scrubs. He rubbed more gel on my stomach before he quickly placed the ultrasound wand on top of my skin, revealing Nora's silhouette on the screen. Her perfect profile projected through the pixels on the monitor, like it had so many times before. But this time her profile was still, like a portrait. Holding my breath, I felt the blood draining from my face. Nora who always moved was motionless.

Maybe she's sleeping? I squinted harder at the screen, searching for signs of life while the doctor moved the wand swiftly over the skin of my belly for vibrations of her pulse. The lack of sound from the speakers and the place in the image on the monitor where her heart in the past would flutter, were both silent and still.

The room spun. I swayed into what seemed like circles. Drifting out of my body and into a tunnel of darkness, I willed myself to resist the shadows enclosing around my vision that warred to pull me away. For a moment, I forgot how to breathe. The doctor kept looking for what seemed like hours, biding time, trying hard to not have to utter the words he and I both knew he was about to say.

"Doctor, what's going on?" Nick pleaded but was ignored. The grave reality of the situation had not settled in for Nick as his face was not yet ghostly white like mine. He hadn't yet accepted the truth that I knew. A mother always knows.

Another jolt of pain, like lightning, contracted through my midsection and around my back with biting intensity. Both my hands clasped the bed rail to brace myself through the abuse. I heard a scream, primal and familiar. The one that woke me from sleep just hours before, but this time the wailing was mine.

Maybe it had been me howling all along.

I held my breath. My brain begged, *Just say it! Get it over with!*

The doctor finally turned his ashen face toward mine. Our eyes locked forebodingly. My breath trembled. He uttered his first words to me, which would be the last I heard as the person I once was.

"I'm sorry." His voice and head both shook. "There's no heartbeat."

In the space of a breath, she was gone.

after

"But when I awake, dear, I was mistaken,

So I hung my head and I cried."

—*Jimmie Davies, "You Are My Sunshine"*

chapter 6

GIVING BIRTH
TO DEATH

"How do we fix this?" Nick asked. He stared at the stillness on the ultrasound screen, thinking our daughter could come back from the dead, because she was not yet born.

"There is nothing we can do. I'm sorry." The doctor had just uttered the words I knew to be true but didn't want to believe. His voice sounded far away and muted, as if I was submerged in water.

At the doctor's reply, Nick's body fell upon my belly where his dead daughter was entombed. I reflexively wrapped my arms around Nick as he wrapped his around Nora inside of me. Pulling his head to my chest between the bump of our dead daughter and my own tears, Nick burrowed his face into my neck and bawled.

Like deer in headlights standing in front of an oncoming car, both the doctor and nurse stared at us silently from above the hospital bed. Not sure what to do, and knowing there was nothing they could do, they waited . . . for what, I wasn't sure. A deep sense of unwarranted anger at the doctor rushed through me, pulling me back into my body and away from whatever darkness I was drifting to. I hated this man, and I had just met him.

Without looking in their direction, I told the doctor and

nurse, "Give us a minute," through tight teeth while I held Nick's weeping and heaving body against mine.

With slumped shoulders and a look of defeat on their faces, they left through the delivery room door carrying the portable ultrasound that couldn't find a heartbeat behind them like dogs dragging their tails between their legs.

"I'm sorry!" I began to croon as Nick cried. Tightening my hands into fists in front of my face, I began searching for answers I could not find and found only blame to give myself instead. "I'm so sorry I couldn't keep her safe. It's my fault!"

Nick lifted himself up from where he laid on my still-covered-in-blue-goo skin that separated us from our never-to-be newborn. Gently pulling my hands away from my face, he locked his gaze with mine. His caring eyes, bloodshot and wet, held a seriousness in their intent. "You didn't do anything to cause this. It's not your fault."

My belly tightened from another contraction coupled with a sudden feeling of disorientation. The room started to get smaller, thinner, and darker as white sparkling stars illuminated the blackness encircling my vision. I blinked hard to bring myself back to the room while I cried, "I should have known something was wrong." My chin trembled as the words tumbled out of my mouth.

"Stop." Nick sat on the small strip of bed next to me and rubbed tears away as he blinked away their wetness. "Just stop," he said, sounding exasperated. He leaned his forehead against mine and cupped both of his hands over my clenched ones. "It's no one's fault."

I nodded vigorously up and down and then back and forth with eyes tightly closed to avoid the present that I wished was a bad dream. I wanted to believe him but didn't. Mothers protected their children. A mother would know if her child died inside her. I was not deserving of the title. Nauseated at the thought, I choked back both tears and bile. I believed that I had failed as a mother. As her mother.

The nice nurse with empathetic eyes and the doctor I dreaded to see sullenly returned to the room. "What happens now?" Nick asked before the staff could speak.

The doctor standing next to me frankly answered, "We deliver."

Flinching, Nick's lips curled back in disgust. His shock-filled face turned multiple shades of gray before his jaw dropped wide open in disbelief once again. "You're not going to give her a C-section?"

They are going to make me labor, only to give birth to a dead baby.

Solemnly shaking his head, the doctor's floppy mop of hair emphasized his answer. "It's not safe." He spoke gently as he held a clipboard clutched against his chest. "Lindsey, you have a temperature of 103 degrees . . . an infection that has caused your baby's death. If we deliver by C-section, it might spread to you. We can't take that risk." His eyes were magnified by his thick glasses, filled with a type of sympathy I wasn't ready to receive. "We will prepare you for labor."

Nick gagged. A hand covered his mouth as he ran to the attached bathroom. I heard him retching. The sound of his hopes and dreams plummeted into the toilet before he flushed away what was supposed to be.

Feeling once again like I was falling down a deep, bottomless well into total darkness, I heard the doctor calling to me from a place far away.

"Lindsey?" he persistently repeated before I had a chance to slip into the seductive nothingness. "Did you hear me?"

I shook my head to reorientate myself to the room.

"We need to prepare you for labor?"

"Okay," I whimpered. Attempting to focus on the doctor's

stoic face, I failed to switch from panic to planning, until I realized the only way I would live through this was to stop the spread of the disease that killed my baby. I had to deliver her. We wouldn't be able to save her life but maybe we could still spare mine. What I heard was that I could die too.

My heart beat wildly in my chest. Death had creeped into my body and stole my baby during the night's quiet darkness. There on the crisp sheets of the cold gurney I could feel her, hovering like a black cloud over the white, fluorescent ceiling lights of the sterile room, readying herself to devour my soul. At that moment, surprisingly, I wasn't scared of Death. For she had already taken from me the one thing a mother could not exist without.

But Nick emerged from the bathroom. Wiping his mouth and taking deep heaving breaths, he slumped against the frame of the door connecting the two rooms, his complexion somehow grimmer than moments before. A look of fear froze on his ashen and pallid face. Spots of water and vomit dotted his gray, zip-up sweatshirt. It was then that the wife part of me was determined to live, even though I wasn't sure I wanted to. Not for me, not for Nora, who they told me was lost to me forever, but for Nick. I wasn't going to leave him alone in this unbearable state of being. It was then I whispered under my breath to Death who stole the soul of my baby and was in my body, attempting to claim mine, "Not today."

Nick took a seat in the chair across from where I lay on the bed and blankly stared at the tile floor, out into his own sea of nothingness.

The kind nurse returned to the room and instructed, "Let me check your cervix."

Moving my attention away from Nick and back to the task at hand. I scooted my bottom to the edge of the bed and the nurse, after inserting her fingers into my vaginal canal, confirmed, "You are four centimeters dilated." Then she held up a long thin piece of metal that looked like a knitting needle.

"I'm going to use this to break your water," she stated before sliding it into my cervix. Upon puncture, rancid, sour-smelling, puke-green-tinted liquid gushed out from between my legs, staining the sheets. Having completed the procedure, she took off her gloves that made a smacking sound against the throbbing silence in the room. Helping me sit up, my naked wet thighs hung over the side of the hospital bed as goosebumps pricked my skin. Lightly touching my shoulder, the nurse caught my gaze and spoke softly to me as if I was a child, "Sweetie, what is your birth plan?"

Plan? I thought. My mouth hung open for more than a moment. *Not this! This was not the plan.* But the words did not come and instead I could only stutter, "I . . . I . . . I don't want to feel."

She thought I meant contractions and childbirth, so she ordered an epidural. But I meant the feeling I couldn't yet describe. My face grew hot at resistance of emotion. My body shook under the surface of my skin, like tiny earthquakes quivering to be released. I pushed them deep down to get through the arduous task of delivering my dead baby.

Shortly after, more nurses and medical staff arrived in the room to roll me out of it. We were transferred off the maternity ward and away from other expectant parents who would get to keep their babies. I was wheeled through the wide and vacant hospital halls on the gurney, Nick followed close behind, and we arrived in another room in a different part of the hospital, where we wouldn't hear the cries of living babies and other new parents wouldn't hear our wails.

Hours passed in a blur. The quick buzzing of an industrial fan set to a beat of electronic beeping became the backdrop of our new hell. White overhead lights blared offensively off pickled-colored walls as blurs of blue-scrub-wearing faceless individuals melted together as one, like fast trains whizzing by a passenger on a station platform. The window, with its plastic blinds a portal to the outside world I was no longer part of, went from dark to light but never did a hint of sunlight shine through. Nick slept during the day, in the uncomfortable vinyl recliner next to my bed as everyone and everything whirled around us like Dorothy inside the eye of a twister. Time stood still but spun out of control all at once.

The nursing shift shuffled. My young, nice nurse was replaced by one in her sixties with short, gray hair and a weathered face. She introduced herself but I could not recall her name, despite her just telling me. This stranger held my hand as Nick slept, and we waited for our families to arrive. While I, according to her, did something referred to as laboring down, but barely felt my body, unsure if this was due to the epidural or my dissociation.

The new nurse spent the time telling me stories. Something about her sister surviving sepsis, which from our conversation and the bags of antibiotics hanging above the bed and flowing through my IV, I gleaned the doctors were worried I might have. She watched the machine that counted my contractions from the pale plastic disc strapped to my belly, where there was supposed to be two monitors, one for my contractions and one for tracking a baby's heartbeat, but only the one needed was in place. She described having shepherded others through the birth of their dead babies. How beautiful their babies were, and how all these unlucky and wounded people were still parents, even though there was no child to show for their claim to the name. She then compassionately explained a photographer was coming to capture the moments that we would spend with our dead daughter. And I thought, *Why would I want pictures of my dead baby?* But I didn't rebuff or refute her request. I didn't have the strength.

"You never have to look at them, dear." She patted my shoulder, taking a momentary pause from monitoring my vitals. "But take them anyway, in case one day you are ready and want to."

The hand of the black-and-white industrial clock, so ordinary and familiar, moved but I could no longer tell time. Minutes had turned to hours, and hours had turned into milliseconds. It was as if I had fallen through a wormhole, sucked into the strange liminal space between death and birth.

As the clock seemed to both spin and stall, our family arrived. They came and went through our room, like warm wind on a damp day. Seemingly out of nowhere, my sister and her husband Zach were suddenly by my side, standing in the spot where the storytelling nurse usually stood.

"I'm so sorry, Lindsey. I'm so sorry," Kristi repeated through shallow breaths as streaks of tears streamed down her cheeks from underneath her magenta-rimmed glasses. She reached to wrap her small, delicate fingers around my swollen ones, cautious not to bump the IV inserted below my thumb, as she choked out, "I love you."

Zach, my sister's sweetheart since high school, six inches taller than her, had hurriedly dressed in a ball cap, sweatpants, and a Chicago Cubs sweatshirt as he stood silently beside her. With his hand on her shoulder, tender tears made their way down his fair-skinned face, while her hand was on mine.

Sometime later or maybe at the same time, Nick's Aunt Susie arrived along with her daughter, Jen, Nick's college-age cousin. They were coincidentally in town from North Dakota for the holiday weekend and stood at the foot of the hospital bed with the same sadness on their face my sister and her husband wore. Susie, with her take-care-by-taking-charge personality, pulled at Nick's arm as I gently pushed him in her direction, hoping he would leave the room to attend to his own needs.

"Maybe go for a walk, or get a cup of coffee," Susie suggested.

But Nick, his hair disheveled with dark bags growing under his eyes, wouldn't budge.

Next, Nick's parents, Barb and Paul walked into the room. I overheard someone say they had made the four-hour drive from Fargo in three hours' time. Paul stoically hugged Nick, giving him a long squeeze of his shoulder before Barb rushed over to be near him. Any composure Nick had managed to muster in the hours since finding out Nora had died melted when his mother wrapped her arms around her grown son, who was once more her baby boy.

Doctors and nurses continued cycling through the revolving door of people circling in and out of the room. A new head doctor on call had taken over for the one I despised. She was older than the previous doctor, probably in her midthirties and petite, with a low, black ponytail that blazed bold against her long white coat. She politely gave us her condolences before stating, "There is a man with his wife in the waiting room claiming he is your father and requesting your medical information."

Her brow narrowed together in frustration. "He is rather persistent about his request. It's against HIPAA for me to tell others about your medical needs."

I smirked, taken aback by the reflex to still choke out a chuckle underneath the mountain of mental anguish sitting on top of my chest. "Is he bald and buff with tattoos that stick out from under rolled-up sleeves of his button-down, flannel shirt and is probably wearing snakeskin cowboy boots?" I asked.

"Yes," she nodded. Her tight features relaxed somewhat at my accurate description. Dad and Mom had arrived from Wisconsin.

"That's my father. It's fine if you update him on things. It might be easier if you do, anyway." I didn't have the strength to discuss with my parents the details of how I had failed to become a parent myself. "After you tell them, will you let them in?"

Within seconds of our conversation, my mom was seated by my side. Bawling uncontrollably, tears ran like rivers down her porcelain and just-beginning-to-wrinkle freckled face. The ball of tissues she held in her hand brushed against my skin when she brought me into her embrace, and the smell of her familiar scent, citrus and hand cream, created a sense of momentary comfort. She tried to speak as she continued crying, but I couldn't understand what she attempted to say. Suddenly and strangely, I sensed myself recoil from her touch. The touch of a mother to a daughter was something Nora would never know.

Dad held Mom in his embrace as his eyes held mine. "I'm so sorry, honey. I don't know what to say." He gently moved Mom to one side of his body, bringing the other toward me. "Just remember I love you. More than anything." He stroked damp hair off the sweaty skin of my forehead I wasn't aware was wet until then. "How are you doing?"

In the presence of my father's concern, my eyes once more filled with water, which had become a bottomless well. Trying to be strong for my struggling parents, I replied, "I'm okay. I can do this." I focused once more on the task of delivering Nora, instead of the thought of her untimely demise, deliberately dissociating from the reality that at birth she would be dead.

Doctor. Dad. Nurses. Nick's parents. Sister. Aunt Susie. They rotated through the room on repeat, like muffled background music I couldn't make out but was comfortingly familiar. Daylight turned to an afternoon winter dusk. Shadows moved across a blank and silent television hanging on the wall of the room. Eventually, the petite and polite doctor returned with another nurse I had not yet met and stood by my bedside.

"It's time," she said. "We are going to deliver your baby now."

I was unaware of what had changed, making it the moment Nora needed to arrive.

As the doctor and two nurses lifted their light-blue surgical masks up to their noses and over their mouths, I turned to Nick, who held my right hand and repeated the words I said on the steps earlier that night. "I am not ready for this."

He nodded and followed the staff's instructions to take a seat on a chair next to the bed. "I'm not, either," he choked out without letting loose from the soft-hearted yet strong grip he had on my hand.

The doctor took her seat at the foot of the bed and scooched her stool uncomfortably close to my spread-apart legs, which framed my view of her face. Her earnest, brown eyes locked with mine above my belly as she reached to pull up the starch white sheet draped over my middle.

Gulping, I held my breath. Images of my baby as a doll-sized, decomposing corpse flashed through my mind. I shivered. The two nurses settled in on each side of me and took up their positions next to my middle, as I wondered, *Will I be repulsed by her? Would I still love her?* I exhaled deeply to expel the frightening thoughts.

A nurse noted, "That's it, Lindsey. Breathe like that."

Each leg was then holstered up and braced back by each nurse while my mind shifted to delusions. *Maybe once delivered, Nora would be fine. We'd prove the doctors and nurses wrong. Their machines were faulty.* My brain attempted to convince my body.

The doctor gave a silent commanding nod in the nurse's direction before I heard one of them turn toward me and instruct, "Push, Lindsey. Push."

I slammed my eyes shut. Blackness was all I wanted to see. It was all that I could feel. I had no idea how to do what they were asking of me, but I gathered strength from a place I didn't know existed deep within and bore down. Every part of me began shaking as droplets of sweat dripped from my forehead where strands of hair stuck to the sides of my face. People yelled directions as my muscles contracted, but I didn't understand their meaning.

I squeezed Nick's cupped hand in mine as hard as I could, my eyes still closed. I heard bodily fluids and blood battle against the suction cup they were using to pull out my baby. Nurses pushed down on my middle in the spot where my ribs met the upward curve that turned into the hill of my stomach. One of them said something about them *helping* with labor because dead babies don't. She dug her elbow into my navel so hard, the pain so sharp, that I bit my lip to fight back my scream.

"Lindsey, look at me." I opened my eyes only at Nick's request, noticing the blood- splattered walls and red-dotted sheet over my chest. "You can do this." He moved his forehead closer to mine. His face was full of concern, but he still attempted to project reassurance that I'm sure he didn't have to give. "We can do this." He was the only thing I could see. Fog surrounded us, blurring the view of everyone and everything else in the room, keeping the horrors of the outside world from creeping in.

"Do you want to touch her head?" the doctor asked. I shook mine in quick jerks in response. The thought that maybe the doctors were wrong and she'd be born breathing kept me pushing. The suction sounds continued to come and go quickly, four, five, six times, maybe more, as if someone was plunging a toilet. The smell of shit mingled with sweat and sanitizer permeated the room.

"One last push," I heard, as the small-framed doctor braced her knee against the bed to leverage herself, pulling back on the suction cup around my baby's head as I pushed. The nurses grunting harmonized with mine as we worked together to labor for a dead baby. Nora's shoulder had caught on my pubic bone, stuck between this world and that of the womb. A final full body contraction caused me to shake uncontrollably. Muscles everywhere within me convulsed as a piercing pain in my pelvis radiated like the universe, expanding throughout my body, with no edges of its end in sight.

The doctor tossed the suction cup to the side, it clanked as it hit the floor before she shoved her hand between my baby's body and mine, tearing open my perineum. My breath became guttural, heavy, and deep. A ring of lightning ripped through me as the doctor continued tearing my skin, and my eyes teared. Shiny bright stars appeared again in my peripheral vision as I teetered on the brink of blacking out.

And then, a sweet release. For a moment, I am free. A lightness lifts me to a place of suspended stillness. There is no noise. No more suction. No more commotion or commands. No movement. No pain. The only sound left in the room is the scream of silence as I wait for the doctor and nurses to be wrong and for a cry that would never come.

chapter 7

HELLO, GOODBYE

"Would you like to hold her?" the doctor asked, before putting a pink knit hat on our daughter's head, covering the suction marks and breaks in her shedding skin where drops of blood descended down the sides of her chalk-white face. Loosely wrapping her in a receiving blanket with the umbilical cord still attached, the doctor approached me with Nora in her arms.

Not ready to see who she was meant to be, but never would, I looked away the moment her 8-pound 12-ounce lifeless body was placed on my chest. Skin to skin, we touched for the first time from the outside when her scent of metallic blood mixed with baby powder found me. I'd waited for this moment for months, not ever imagining it would be like this. Afraid to look down and see that the baby I held in a cream-colored blanket in the nook of my arm was a corpse. For I still held onto a dissociated hope that the doctors were wrong.

Breathless. I didn't think I could ever breathe again, but then my lungs filled with air while hers remained empty. *This is not how it was supposed to be,* I repeated in my mind. Squinting my already-shut eyes tighter together, I inhaled deeply one more time before summoning the courage to turn my gaze toward her.

Don't look. You'll never be able to go back, I screamed inside my mind. But on exhale, I opened my eyes and everything else faded away. The sound of the machines beeping disappeared, and the feeling of the doctor inserting stitches departed. I didn't mind that my skin was soaked with sweat and drenched in the dampness of bodily fluids. I could no longer smell the stench of antiseptic mixed with my blood that had spewed all over the floor or notice that Nick had stepped away from the hospital bed, his hand held over his mouth as tears streamed down his face.

All I could see was her.

In the place where seconds ago I could not look, I found myself unable to look away, mesmerized by my daughter. She was a beautiful baby, with long brown eyelashes and big dark black lips. I would never know the sound of her coo or the color of her eyes, as they would never open, and I couldn't bear to peek because I wanted to remember her like this. For even in death, she was stunning. Her face was heart-shaped and white like winter. She had ten fingers and ten toes perfectly in place. Her soft-to-the-touch skin was a shade of gray, like when chimney smoke and ash mix on a snowy night, and it was even still somewhat warm, as I was told my body had kept hers from becoming cool.

"Nick, look! She's perfect!" I said joyfully through conflicted tears that flooded and fogged up my glasses, convincing myself for a brief second she was alive. Never had I experienced love like this, and I did not want it to slip away.

Wanting with everything in my being to pretend her paleness was like Snow White, and she was just asleep like Sleeping Beauty. But the kiss I placed on her stony forehead would not make her wake. Every passing second her body without breath became more tepid to my touch. But at that beautifully cruel moment, I did not notice, because all I could see was her brilliance.

Nick moved meekly toward the two of us, gathering up his own courage to inch onto the bed. The nurse asked if he wanted to cut the umbilical cord, but he shook his head. His eyes were fixed on his dead daughter, who would forever be a dream never to come true. Reaching his two fingers toward the top of Nora's receiving blanket, he gently pulled back the fabric from her face to meet her for the first time.

"She is beautiful," Nick could barely breathe out as his voice trembled. Lifting a finger, he softly brushed her pale cheek with the back of his hand and then patted a patch of her wispy chocolate-colored hair, like his, that peeked out from under the pink, knit cap she wore.

"She's so perfect!" I repeated, wanting to somehow desperately hang onto the moment of delusion a little longer. "Don't you think she is perfect?" I asked.

I don't remember if Nick ever answered. I became distracted by a drop of red blood that dripped out of her nose, contrasting brightly against her ghostly shaded skin. I was watching our future slip away.

Time once again stood still, while at the same time everything was morphing in form. She and I were no longer one, and yet somehow intertwined as I held her breathless body against my breathing one.

A new nurse entered the room. She smiled at me and introduced herself. "Would you like to dress your daughter?" she asked as she stood above Nick and I seated on the bed with Nora cradled in my arms. "You could use the clothes you brought with you." She quickly glanced toward our packed hospital bag in the corner of the room. "Or ones that we have?"

Consumed by shock and sorrow, I shook my head to silently decline the offer to dress her.

"Would it be okay if I did it then?" The nurse held out her arms. "I'll bring her right back." She smiled for reassurance. "I promise."

I silently nodded in agreement as I passed my perfect but dead daughter into her hands.

Gently cradling my baby against her chest, she asked before walking away, "What is her name?"

Nick rubbed my back as I looked at him before I whispered, "Nora."

The nurse gulped back her own sadness. A small quiver crept across her lip before she responded, "That's a beautiful name."

Nick and I clung to each other while we watched from a few feet away as the nurse dipped and dampened a washcloth in a small basin of water. Drops of water dripped back into the bowl as she squeezed it before she gently sponged Nora's delicate and decaying skin.

The nurse silently sobbed as she softly sang to our dead daughter, her own made-up song. "You're beautiful, sweet baby girl Nora. What a beautiful baby you are."

Tears dotted the nurse's face as she delicately dressed Nora in a soft pink onesie. She wrapped her again in the receiving blanket she was placed in after birth, with the kind of care one would bestow on their own newborn. Later I learned she had recently had a baby, too. A daughter. Also named Nora.

She then placed a snuggly wrapped Nora back into my arms. "You can stay with her as long as you like." I nodded, knowing that the lifetime I had imagined was not what was implied. "Do you want me to send in your family or would you like to go get them?" She asked us both but looked at Nick. "They are anxiously waiting in the hall to see you all."

"If you are ready, I can get everyone." Nick gently brushed Nora's cool forehead before he placed a long kiss on mine.

Holding Nora and feeling her weight once again heavy on my chest, I shut my eyes. These fleeting moments with her would soon end. I whispered, "Okay."

Nora and I were alone together for the first and last time. Swaddled in the receiving blanket and dressed in a fleece onesie, she deceivingly felt warm against my skin. I deliberately forgot my dream of her coming home would not come true. Lifting my arms with her in them, I bent forward to kiss her cool head. "I'm so sorry." I whispered into her ear that could not hear me. "I'm sorry that I didn't know."

The room was silent except for my sniffling when Nick returned. He held the door for our family to file in. My mother and father entered first and stood by my side. Kristi and Zach followed and fell in line next to my parents, starting an arch around my hospital bed. Next, Aunt Susie and Cousin Jen stood at my feet, and Nick's parents, Barb and Paul, completed the half circle of love that had risen like the morning sun around us. Nick took his seat next to me in the open spot on the bed and fidgeted with Nora's receiving blanket so our family could see her face. "Lindsey, tell them her name."

It was then my dream-like state was broken. Our dead daughter suddenly became heavy in my hands. My arms lost tension as I sobbed and shook, realizing our family didn't know her name because this was supposed to be the moment when we had planned for them to say hello, not goodbye to her.

Instead of announcing her name, I clutched Nora closer to my caved-in chest and cried, "She feels so good," knowing I couldn't keep her. Barb covered her mouth, and Mom's eyes went wide with pain as she witnessed my agony. Kristi sniffled, and Susie grabbed her grown daughter's hand. Uncertain of what to say, everyone remained silent.

Nick rubbed my back and shushed in my ear, "It's okay. Take your time."

I breathed deeply through my stuffed-up nose. With the back of my hand, I wiped away snot mixed with tears from above my mouth before I finally spoke. "Her name is Norine Kelly Henke." My chest quivered as I exhaled. "We were planning on calling her Nora."

WHEN SKIES ARE GRAY

At the announcement of her name, we heard a collective sigh and an *awww* by our family. Barb wept gently. Nora's middle name was her maiden one. My mother openly sobbed.

"Would you like to hold her?" Nick asked everyone, and my mother rushed to the front of the line. She bent forward with outstretched and eager arms to pick up her first grandchild, and I released Nora into my mother's hands. A ritual and a rite of passage I'm sure most dream about was somehow both a beautiful and brutal moment for us both.

Nora was tenderly passed from one family member's arms into the next. My father only held her momentarily. He had one eye breathing in Nora's beauty and the other firmly fixed on me. The gentle hands of my sister bravely brushed the sides of Nora's white face.

Aunt Susie swayed with Nora in her arms and said, "Spend as much time with her as you can. Rock her. Dress her. Bathe her. Sing to her. Make a lifetime of memories in moments."

Nick and I nodded at her suggestion as Nora was passed to the next loved one in line waiting to meet her.

Tears from each family member fell onto Nora's empty body. Collective wet droplets, like a rain-spotted street accumulated on her pale-pink fleece—gathered from aunts and uncles, grandmas and grandpas not to be. A chorus of sniffles resounded throughout the room. Nora completed her cycle through the circle of loved ones with my father-in-law. I'd never seen him waver in his calm demeanor until that day when a silent tear tumbled down his cheek. My mother ran next to Paul to hold Nora one last time.

The afternoon turned to dusk and then darkness. The city lamplight shimmered into the hospital window through the plastic blinds creating stripped shadows across the tile floor. Nick, Nora, and I waited for a photographer from southern Minnesota to arrive, about an hour and half away. It was said she drove through a snowstorm in negative temperatures to take pictures of our deceased baby, who as the minutes passed, was looking more and more like winter herself.

The photographer carried her camera by a large strap around her neck while holding the lens in her hand when the nurse escorted her into the room. Immediately, she started snapping photos. Nick, Nora, and I as a family of three sat on the hospital bed with the sound of her lens clicking as it captured our only moments together. The pictures the photographer took would be given to us in black-and-white, which was how my memories would be of those moments . . . no longer in color but in different shades of gray. Nora's dark lips kept falling open into an oval shape, and the photographer gently attempted but failed to push her chin back into place for the last portrait. No matter how much I wanted to believe Nora looked like any other newborn, she was just a shell of herself.

In the few hours that had passed since her birth, her dark-shaded lips had become even darker, and the once-warm receiving blanket no longer kept the cruelness of her coolness at bay. Her icy-cold body had let go of all the heat from mine. I couldn't bear to hold her any longer. I couldn't do all the things Susie said. To rock her. To sing to her. To make a lifetime of memories in moments.

We turned our short hello into a forever goodbye. Nick placed a kiss on her cold forehead and so did I. I then handed Nora into the arms of the nurse with a daughter by the same name. I was giving my baby back to the space from which she came . . . not to my womb but the molecules of the universe she was made from. The nurse placed Nora in the bassinet beside the bed and said, "I can bring her back to your room whenever you like."

But never again would we see Nora in her earthly form.

When the nurse rolled the bassinet into the hallway, I heard the grandmothers pleading, "Where are you taking her?" They still somehow believed Nora would be going home, instead of being brought to the morgue.

When the door closed, the eruption of emotions I had been keeping at bay, like bubbling lava under my skin, let loose. I no longer tried wiping tears away as an animalistic howl roared out of my chest. I rocked back and forth on the bed. Nick held me in his arms as we swayed together in indescribable sadness. Finally, giving into exhaustion, I slipped into the darkness of a dreamless sleep.

chapter 8

SUPPOSED TO

Between the world we drift to each night and the one where we wake, I still felt her. A temporary amnesia set in my body and in "that place between sleep and awake," as Tinkerbell describes to Peter Pan, "that place where you still remember dreaming," Nora lived inside of me, no longer as the symbiotic creatures we used to be of mother and child, but as a felt sense—as if she encompassed my whole being and was no longer confined to my womb.

Floating above myself, I saw my body below, collapsed onto Nick's chest in the hospital bed, lingering longer in that liminal space, where momentarily I was able to catch my breath. Before my eyes fully opened, I basked in the glory of not knowing.

A soft brush of my cheek resurrected my soul from that place of relief and brought me back into my broken body, cradled in my husband's arms. Prickles swept over my skin. With my weight upon his, Nick caressed my face, like he would have done to soothe her. His fatherly gestures with nowhere to go he mournfully passed along to me. A white light beamed through my closed eyes, encompassing us, as if we were aglow. Upon opening them, it felt like I was being reborn. The luminous rays faded away to bring me back to my husband on earth.

The aches of delivering Nora's shell of a self slowly echoed throughout my body. The epidural had worn off in the night while

I slept. With any slight movement, everything from my waist down radiated with pain, and my skin stank of illness mixed with antiseptic. I slowly sat up, unconsciously bringing my hand to my belly. My once round, basketball-sized stomach now looked like a deflated balloon. Empty inside.

I desperately wanted to drift off again into the expanse of nothingness and vacate this world for another where Nora might reside. I wished, for a moment, that I, too, could have perished, so I could forget that the world was forever broken, I was forever broken, and she was dead.

We were visited by the hospital social worker, a young woman barely a college graduate, who briefly gave us her condolences and left us with a blue, file folder packet of a kind of *What to Expect When You Are No Longer Expecting Because Your Baby Died.* Inside were pamphlets for funeral homes, therapists, and a glossy brochure for a grief retreat with happy-again people in its pictures.

"Why would anyone want to go to a grief retreat?" I wondered out loud to Nick. I rolled over, turned my back toward him, and pulled the fresh hospital sheet up to my shoulder as he flipped through the paperwork with our new life instructions inside.

Later that afternoon, a gray-haired doctor with creases in the corners of her eyes sat next to me on a corner of the bed and explained Nora's death was a fluke. I shut my eyes to focus on her words. The results weren't back, but they believed it was an infection, named chorioamnionitis. A one-in-a-million chance occurrence. We had won the shitty-luck lottery, and bacteria had made it through a microscopic tear in the fetal membranes, contaminating the one place Nora was supposed to remain safe.

Opening my eyes, I asked, "If we try to have another child, will this happen again?" My heart hurt as I uttered this out loud. *Try again* . . . as if we struck out at home plate and would just simply get another swing at parenthood, and somehow everything would be okay.

She replied with an attempt at a soothing tone, "I wasn't going to mention this until you were ready. Yes, you can still have children, but unfortunately, having one stillbirth increases your chances of having another." She placed her hand on my knee. "Do you have any more questions?"

Swallowing hard, I bit my lip to hold back tears, summoning the courage to ask the one question I had been fearing to hear the answer to since I first learned Nora died. "Did I do something wrong?"

Nick quickly came to my bedside, swooped his arm around my back and brought me in tight to his torso, "Lindsey, stop it! This is not your fault."

Pausing for a moment to gather her thoughts, the doctor took her glasses off and rested them upon her chest where they hung by a black lanyard around her neck. "No. Your husband is right. You didn't do anything wrong."

I'm her mother! Isn't it my job to protect her? To bring her into this world alive, not dead? "Then why did my body do this?" I asked.

With sympathetic authority, the doctor made her case to counter my doubts. "Your body was trying to save you. It's the body's job to get rid of the infection. To do that you needed to deliver your baby."

I was unable to find solace in her words. If I didn't do something tangibly wrong, maybe it was something karmically wrong. Was it the joke I made to coworkers a week ago when they noticed I no longer fit into my maternity slacks? I had worn yoga pants and sandals to therapy sessions during a December snowstorm.

"How is pregnancy going?" two fellow therapists asked while we were in the break room.

"I've kept her alive so far," I quipped. It must have been the kiss-of-death reply.

Patting my knee, the doctor grabbed my hand and held my gaze. She was careful with the words she chose next, not knowing her answer would only cause me more despair. "Your body did what it's supposed to do." But we both knew it wasn't supposed to be like this.

We were discharged that evening. The next day we were supposed to be arriving at the hospital for our scheduled induction to deliver our New Year's baby, not leaving on New Year's Eve without one. Nick and I waited for the elevator when another couple approached.

Their eyes beamed with delight. The man, with an upturned face, carried a balloon attached to a car seat with a newborn inside that read, "It's a girl!" The glowing woman leaned down to tuck a blanket below her baby's chin. I wanted so badly to stop staring, but I couldn't look away from what might have been.

The elevator doors opened, and the happy couple waited for the occupants inside to exit. I could have imagined it, but another couple with a very pregnant wife who appeared to be in labor stepped out before they could step in. The future and past versions of these couples had come face-to-face with each other as they exchanged a knowing smile between them, like a secret handshake Nick and I had not been given. I viewed this event as a bystander, as if I was an extra in their play, and not the protagonist of my own. These main characters were cheerfully in their own little world, not noticing our puffy eyes, slumped stances, or empty arms.

The couple who got to keep their baby held the door of the elevator for us. I stood there frozen, unable to feel my legs, even as my mind willed them to move. My eyes fixated on their breathing, baby girl.

"That's how it's supposed to be," I whispered to myself. Nick signaled to the couple that we would wait for the next elevator.

A bitter breeze assaulted my face when we exited the elevator and walked out the double doors of the hospital and into the parking lot. Crisp icy air mingled with the smells of a frozen city. Upon seeing our car, my chest tightened. Panicked, my breath became quick, recalling the empty car seat inside where Nora was supposed to be.

I cautiously climbed in, trying to find a position to sit that wouldn't cause pain for my perineal stitches. I reached behind me for my seatbelt without looking over my shoulder. How could we have been so presumptuous to believe that when we left the hospital, we would bring home a baby? We had driven with the car seat installed weeks before Nora's arrival, innocently assuming we were impervious to fate's wheel of misfortunes. I looked ahead through the frosted windshield, fearful to look behind.

Nick fiddled with the heater and noticed the rigidness of my stare. Touching my hand, he reassured me, "It's not there."

Even though I knew what he was referring to, I asked to be sure. "What's not there?"

"The car seat. Kristi and Zach took it out."

Closing my eyes, I let my held breath release.

When we arrived home, the house was dark. The silent stillness of the delivery room had carried over into our home. Life was now broken into two parts: *before* we left for the hospital and *after* we arrived, only to be told she had died. And in the *after*, all I could see, feel, and know was darkness. Nick's parents, who agreed to stay at our place to take care of George while we were away, had left the Christmas tree lights on for our arrival. Its red, green, and white twinkle lights cast an eerie glow upon the walls, reminiscent of a candle illuminating a tomb.

I walked by the tree and down the hallway that led past Nora's room and to ours. The door to her nursery was still shut. Why did I close the door? Did I somehow know we wouldn't need to open it again because she was already dead inside of me? I shook away the memory of foolishly speaking to her things before we left for the hospital, telling them she would soon be there. Now, behind the door awaited a nursery Nora would never use.

Diverting my eyes, I passed by her bedroom and focused on making it into ours. I was so tired, a kind of exhaustion I had never experienced before. Muscles I didn't know I had ached from birthing Nora, while every cell of my body yearned to hold her. My arms wept with a molecular sadness that settled into my DNA.

I threw myself on the bed. Collapsing onto the mattress, I was aware of my swollen but empty belly. Slowly, I pulled back the freshly-washed quilt that smelled of fabric softener my mother-in-law had laundered, revealing the clean white linens I had slept on a night ago. Suddenly, my hands shook, realizing on my side of the bed, between those sheets, Nora had been alive for the last time, nestled inside of me. It was also the place Nick and I innocently slept as she died. I let the sheet fall from between my fingers. Feeling lightheaded and nauseous, I stood up and backed away from what was supposed to be my side of the bed and chose the pillows on Nick's half to settle into.

We fell asleep to *Family Guy* reruns, drifting off into my own darkness in between the sheets where she died. Over the next few weeks, Nick turned on the television nightly in hopes of turning off his mind. He did not want to be alone with his thoughts. I did not want to let go of mine, clinging to them for fragments of her.

Sleeping made the pain stop, even though I wanted nothing more than to find her in my dreams. In the weeks ahead, I'd read books and articles about how to let your loved one visit you while you slumber with the intention to penetrate the veil between the living and the dead. I didn't dream of Nora that first night home after her death, but in the years that followed, I continued to hope, in vain, that she would come to me in my dreams.

✔✔✔

The next morning, I woke to Nick softly kissing my forehead. Not wanting to wake, I pretended to be asleep even though I felt rested. I was supposed to be exhausted from night nursing a newborn every few hours not unfatigued. The haunting silence of our house hurt my ears. My body was numb, its senses discombobulated as if I could see sound and hear sight.

Nick persisted and drew the curtains open. An intrusive light beat at my eyes. Looking away, I squinted, wondering how the sun did not get the message that her cherry brightness no longer fit my feelings of defeat. My depressive state craved drearier days. It was the morning of New Year's, the day we were supposed to be induced with Nora.

Sighing, I sat up in bed. "What time will everyone be here?"

Nick had arranged for both our parents, Kristi, and Zach to come over for our family Christmas we had postponed to celebrate the holiday with Nora.

Nick rubbed my shoulder and replied, "This evening." He handed me a glass of water, two Tylenol, and a pain medication my doctor prescribed. "Take this."

Picking up the pills from the palm of his open hand, I gulped them down with a glass of water.

Nick informed me of my daily schedule—what medications to take, when it was time to eat, and which visitors were to be expected. It was his way of believing he could keep me from falling into a deep depression that he knew visited more than once in the years before we met. I didn't tell him it would likely happen no matter what precautions he took.

"Are we opening presents today?" I asked, remembering the gifts I had specially made for each family member. A necklace with an engraved pendant that said, "Grandma" for my mom. A keychain that read, "Grandpa" for my dad and Nick's, and a bracelet engraved with, "Awesome Aunt" for my sister. Each gift honored a family member's new role in what was supposed to be Nora's long-lived life. I sighed for a second time and said, "It's time."

"It's time for what?" Nick asked, looking confused as he sat on the edge of the bed, still in his pajama pants and sweatshirt.

"It's time for me to give you your last Christmas gift. The one from Nora and me."

Nick looked away and into his lap, trying to hide his sadness.

"Are you ready?"

"I guess," he sighed.

There is a lot of sighing in grief. I'd later learn it's a common physical symptom of the bereaved. The grief-stricken and those who witness their mourning report this weird occurrence in the grieving. It's as if each sigh is a resistant surrender into the present that wasn't supposed to be.

"It's downstairs in your stocking. I can go get it." Pushing my hands against the mattress, I tried to pull myself out of bed, wincing from a violent jolt of pain palpitating my groin.

Nick stood up and stopped me. "Stay there. I'll get it. You need to rest." He left the room briefly and quickly returned with a tiny box wrapped in red-and-white candy cane Christmas paper.

With the gift in hand, he crawled into bed next to me, where our bodies touched under the covers. Craving closeness, we clung to each other as our only life rafts, like drowning swimmers in the middle of the sea. We took every opportunity to hold each other and hug each other, trying desperately to fill the void of parental affection we were supposed to be lavishing upon Nora with continual contact from each other.

Nick paused before opening the box. Tears slowly creeped into the corners of his eyes. Watching him hurt agonized me more than my own pain, for I had caused his. "I'm sorry she's not here to give it to you." I was sorry. Sorry that he never got to hold her while she was alive. Sorry that I could not give him the one thing a wife was supposed to be able to give her husband. Sorry that I could not keep our child safe. Sorry that I failed as a mother. I was sorry for so many things that I did not say out loud.

He took a deep breath and delicately unwrapped the decorative paper from around the box. Hesitantly, he opened the gift, as if it was his own Pandora's box of emotions he held in his hands, afraid if he let them out, he could never put them back in. With the wrapping paper gone, he gently held the tiny package between his fingers. His left hand moved the lid away as his right hand reached for the key chain, a brass military man's dog tag at the bottom of the box. Lifting the gift to eye level, he read the inscription I had engraved.

Husband
Father
Hero

Love,
Wife & Daughter

The well of tears that waited in the wings spilled over his cheeks and sobs exploded from his lungs. He hung his head in his hands with the key chain clenched in his fist. I wrapped my arms around him, and we melted into each other once again. We were supposed to be holding her, but we held each other instead as we clung to what little memories we had of a never-lived life.

The funeral home smelled of day-old flowers. I took a seat on an office chair and pulled myself up to a conference table in a small private room. I glanced at Nick seated next to me. He wore a black peacoat and light-blue button-up shirt with jeans as if he was attending a casual business meeting and not planning his dead daughter's funeral. He flashed a forced smile in my direction through exhausted eyes with dark circles under them. Seeing Nick's grief grow overnight on his face, I wondered how I must have looked in my chunky gray sweater over leggings with wet hair and no makeup.

I had no idea what new parents did in the first few days of a living baby's life. I never let myself think that far ahead. Why was that? I wondered. However, I did know new parents were not supposed to be sitting across from an elderly woman, who looked like Betty White but wasn't funny. Her name tag under her brooch read, "Patricia, Funeral Home Director." She helped us choose a death announcement and celebration of life ceremony program more suited for someone who had taken a breath in this world.

Flipping to the last page of a three-ring binder, Patricia pointed to examples of funeral services programs with teddy bears and cradles on them. They were tucked away in the back of the book in hopes that most of the grieving who visited her establishment wouldn't be burdened with knowing their grief could be worse. Other bereaved people usually got more time with those they mourned. The days printed on their longed-for-loved-one's program would have years represented in the dash between the dates instead of just one day, like Nora's did.

Is Nora's date a birth date or a death date? You must be alive to be born, right? Legally we never received a birth certificate, only a certificate of stillbirth, so if it's not a birth date printed on her program, then was it a death date without a date of birth? It is all very confusing when someone dies before they live. I pointed to the least ugly program for Nora's ceremony and closed the binder.

"Who would you like to officiate your service?" Patricia politely asked.

"We aren't religious," I replied.

After the Golden Girl look-alike recommended a non-faith-based officiant to facilitate Nora's ceremony, Nick requested a religious prayer be included in our secular service, just in case—a kind of CYA with God.

We were then taken to a room filled with urns. The infant ones were kept in a small, not hidden but not noticeable, section in the corner. There was a plastic white one, a wooden one with a floral cross, and a bronze metal one with an ugly white ceramic teddy bear on the front. Nick, worried about whether Nora would be warm in her final resting place, voted no to the plastic urn, as he thought it wasn't insulated enough. And as a nonbeliever, I couldn't put my daughter's ashes into a box labeled with an ideology I didn't buy into. I pointed to the only other option left on the shelf.

"We'll take that one." None of it made a difference as neither of our needs made logical sense. Nora would soon be reduced to particles of dust and would not care what her urn looked like, or if it was comfortable.

But bereft parents do and think strange things in their final and only acts left in parenting their children. Which meant the ugly bronze box with its white ceramic teddy bear would be our daughter's forever home.

"What would you like engraved on her urn?" was a question I was asked that baby books didn't prepare me to answer.

"Her name. Just her name," I replied. Leaving the confusing date off her urn would take away having to make sense out of it.

Exhausted, I was ready to leave when I noticed a silver necklace with a tiny hand etched into a pendant displayed on the hutch in the hallway. Standing in front of the oak sideboard, I ran my fingertips over the small yet unique handprint inside the pendant. "Is this someone's actual handprint?"

Patricia nodded with her tightly-curled white hair bobbing.

Having nothing left of Nora to hold, I suddenly needed the necklace. Liking the idea of carrying a unique piece of her next to my heart, linking us in some way, "Can I get one with Nora's footprint?"

Again, nodding, Patricia reached for the brochure by the display. "What type of metal would you like?"

I looked to Nick since he tended toward the frugal side.

"You can get whichever one you want," he said softly.

I wanted the white gold. "It's almost a thousand dollars?" I asked, my fingers touching my parted lips as I looked at the price.

"Let's get it." Pulling out his credit card from his wallet, he handed it to Patricia. In the wake of death, money was no longer a concern for Nick. It now seemed empty and meaningless, for it couldn't buy back our baby.

"One more thing before you go," Patricia interjected as we made our way toward the front door. "I wanted to let you know, she's here." She pointed to a room down a short hallway. "You can see her."

The quickening pulse in my chest grew louder in my ears. *See her? Do I want to see her?* Oh, how I ached to see her. I wanted to see her as she clasped her hand around my finger, as her eyes opened and looked into mine. I wanted to brush my fingers against her dark, wispy hair one more time. I wanted to feel her warm body next to my breast.

But I shook my head because I didn't want to see her blue face with even darker black lips than before. I didn't want to run my hands over her cold, tiny body laid frozen on a stainless-steel table. But mostly, I didn't want to feel the pain of having to be separated from her again.

"Love knows not its own depth until the hour of separation," Kahlil Gibran wrote in the *Prophet*.

I never wanted to love that much again.

When we returned home, instead of sharing her birth on Facebook, we announced her death. Our parents insisted on putting an obituary in the local paper, but we informed them that was not how our generation announced milestones in life. I found love online. I found my job online. We found our house online. We announced our pregnancy online. It only made sense to announce death online, too.

Then, in true millennial fashion, I turned to Google instead of God for my answers. During the sleepless nights, or long, drawn-out days shortly after her death, I was glued to my devices. Obsessively, I would type, "Why did *my* baby die?" into the search engine of my phone or computer while lying on the couch or in bed in my pajamas, under a blanket and with a bag of ice between my legs to soothe my swollen vagina. Closing my eyes after pressing enter, I waited for a response to pop up, like I did in my youth with a Magic 8 Ball after shaking it, hoping to get answers to my questions. But my Magic 8 ball was broken because Google could not provide any explanations to the questions of, "Why Nora? Why me? Why us?"

My best friend from high school, Staci, who lived down the country road from me during childhood, called one evening early after Nora's death.

"I didn't know this could happen. That babies could still die before they are born." My friend from before we knew about the birds and the bees continued to ponder. "I thought that only happened in the 1800s. Not nowadays, with today's medicine."

Staci's wondering on our phone call gave me an idea. If Google couldn't give me an answer to my existential question, then maybe WebMD would be able to answer my medical ones. I grabbed my laptop from under my bed where I sat above it. She was right, or so I thought. Today's medicine was supposed to be able to keep people alive, especially before they had a chance to live. This time, I was more specific in asking my Magic 8 Ball questions. My fingers floated over the keys to find WebMD and typed into its search bar, "chorioamnionitis," which only led me to learn that Nora *could* have lived. Some babies don't die from an intrauterine infection; their mother's body saves them. It starts labor or gives the mother a sign that something was wrong.

Angry, I slammed shut my computer, questioning WebMD's stupid answer. My body didn't give me any signs. I closed my eyes and tried remembering back to that evening. But what if it did? Maybe, if I'd gone in earlier that night, when I noticed her movements had slowed down, I could have saved her? Falling forward over the pillow in my lap that had propped up my computer, I curled into the fetal position and cried. With each sob, my shoulders heaved with a heaviness I feared I would forever carry.

The week following Nora's death, our parents took turns taking care of us. They drifted in and out of the house like I drifted in and out of the nightmare. Nick's parents prepared our home for our return from the hospital. They washed dishes that weren't dirty and shoveled snow off the already-salted sidewalk before they left for North Dakota to pick up Nick's twelve-year-old niece, Hannah, for the funeral the following Saturday.

My mother and father stayed with us after Nick's parents left. In the mornings, I would wake to the sound of Dad vacuuming stairs that didn't display a speck of dirt and smell Mom cooking scrambled eggs that I didn't have the appetite to eat. She watched me with anxious eyes as I only wandered from the bedroom to the couch where I cuddled up under a blanket and continued searching the internet for answers.

Dad put words to his worry, asking, "Have you eaten today?" or "How did you sleep?" Their protective parental instincts took hold of them as it must naturally do in dire times. I guess I wouldn't know since I was no longer a mom. At least I didn't think I was. *How can one be a mom if there is no child to mother?*

On one of those afternoons, my mother was behind the master bathroom door, composing herself after I had just finished showing both my parents pictures of Nora taken after her birth. The photographer had emailed us the edited photos in time for tomorrow's funeral. I was so glad we listened to the nurse who insisted we take the pictures. She was right. With each photo I shared with my parents, I was able to be Nora's mom, and they could be her grandparents, like we were supposed to be.

"She is beautiful," my father said. We sat on my bed, and he wrapped one arm around my shoulder while looking at a photo of Nora. My head laid on his chest like the little girl I once was. The scent of his familiar, musky cologne brought me a moment of comfort, reminding me of when I was a child and life seemed less hard.

Silently, he kissed my forehead as I sniffled. Both of us were still while looking at Nora's pale face glowing from the computer screen on my lap when he whispered in my ear, "I would have traded places with her, you know. For you. For Nora."

I didn't see a tear in his eyes, but they welled in mine.

For a moment, I floated back to being his baby and let my little-girl self linger in his embrace. "Thank you, Daddy. I know."

Later that evening, I woke under a blanket in front of the fireplace with Georgie snuggled into the bent part of my knees. I heard Nick chopping vegetables for a side salad to the lasagna he was warming up, dropped off by considerate neighbors and friends. My groggy eyes opened to crackling orange-and-yellow ribboned flames dancing across smoke-stained bricks, burning the logs inside to ash and dust. The words from the funeral home director, "You can see her," played in my mind. And I did see Nora, with her button nose, heart-shaped face, and naked baby body. Burning in the fire.

I began trembling. Rocking back and forth, I clutched my blanket and fixated on the flames. *What have we done? I must see her. Why did I recoil when given the opportunity to see her?* Now Nora's body was burning. She was burning. She was ash and dust. Never again would I see Nora in the form that I made her.

I yelled to Nick, "When is Nora being cremated?" *Maybe we can see her again? I must see her. One more time.*

"The funeral is tomorrow. It probably already happened." Nick found me in a ball of panic near the hearth on the carpeted floor.

Maybe it's happening now? Nora may be letting me know she was leaving this world for good. My voice quivered when I looked up toward Nick kneeling above me. "Do you think it's already done?"

Softly rubbing my back in circles, he whispered, "Yeah, I do."

My chest became heavy, rising and falling quickly as I struggled to breathe. If I didn't feel her dying inside of me, I wouldn't be able to feel her being refashioned into dust, either. Helpless to the pressure building in my lungs, I threw myself back onto the blanket in front of the fire and cried. Animalistic sobs roared out of me from a place deep within. I heard Nick sniffle as he caressed my shoulders. My mind raced with questions of injustice and pleas of acquittal to Mother Nature, God, the Universe, whoever would listen. *Why did you take her from me? It's not supposed to be this way. She's supposed to be here. In my arms. Please, just give her back and wake me from this nightmare.*

chapter 9

INVISIBLE MOTHER

On Saturday morning, five days after Nora died, I woke in bed in the same spot where, a week ago, Nick and I professed to each other we were the happiest we had ever been. Six days ago, it was the place where Death stole Nora from me silently as I slept. How quickly things can change. Or as Joan Didion wrote in *The Year of Magical Thinking*, "Life changes fast. Life changes in the instant. The ordinary instant." Our lives . . . altered in the space of a breath never taken.

Sighing deeply, I rolled out of bed and noticed my breasts were painfully engorged under my nightgown and had grown two sizes overnight. I called my doctor's office for advice. The nurse recommended I bind my breasts in the tightest sports bra I could find to help cease milk production. My body was playing another cruel trick on me—lactating. My body, after failing to protect my baby, still foolishly thought it was a mother. The nurse said something about expecting a letdown, but thankfully that had not happened. Not owning a sports bra that fit the new size my breasts had become, Nick and I took a trip to Target to pick one up and print off Nora's photos for her funeral.

Entering Target, we made our way to the photo kiosk next

to the return desk in the front of the store. Nick and I waited for Nora's black-and-white pictures to print in seconds as I wondered what the young, twenty-something store clerk dressed in a red-collared shirt would say if we hadn't taken all the tags off Nora's things and tried to return them.

"Was there something wrong with your purchase?"

"No, it's just that dead babies don't need bottles." How would the clerk respond? Maybe he'd already learned the hard way not to ask questions for returns on newborn items.

Watching photos of my pale and lifeless baby flop onto the kiosk's tray, a baby started to cry. The skin around my nipples became cold. Looking down at my chest, I noticed my shirt was damp. Two wet spots had grown over my nipples expanding outward on the fabric of my thin sweater. The letdown. I cursed myself for having left my coat in the car and crossed my arms over my chest as if I were naked and someone had walked in on me while stepping out of the shower.

Panicked, I said to Nick who was putting the only photos we would ever take of Nora in an envelope and said, "We need to go, now!"

Nick stood still, startled by my adamant request and awkward body contortion.

"Can I have the keys, please? I'll wait in the car."

He reached into his pocket, and I quickly snatched the key ring from his hand, ignoring his look of frustration, and raced out the store's sliding glass doors. Slipping into the passenger's seat, a part of me felt guilty for leaving Nick to do the difficult job of purchasing our dead baby's photos by himself, but I couldn't handle the sudden sadness dripping from my breasts.

Two hours before her funeral, I was curled up in bed with sulfur-smelling cabbage leaves in between my new sports bra and leaky breasts. The house bustled with people outside my bedroom door. I had told everyone I was taking a nap before the funeral, when the truth was, I was hiding from them and trying to find her, searching for Nora in the place where I felt her move for the last time.

Lying on Nick's side of the bed, I willed myself to remember the final moments of her life. With my eyes closed and hands on my loose and empty middle, I attempted to remember the night before she died. She had moved that evening—I know she did. But now I questioned if her movements were even real. They were so subtle and soft, not like her usual strong shifts. Maybe she was sick when I thought she was moving? What kind of mother doesn't know when her baby is dying inside her? *The kind that doesn't deserve to be a mother.*

A flutter moved within my vacant womb, as if Nora was kicking me, still there, letting me know she was okay. But rubbing my hand back and forth over the squishy skin of my deflated belly, I was reminded Nora was gone. A phantom kick must have vibrated through the muscle memory in my pelvis. My body still hoped we had a chance at being her mother.

With my eyes and my hands on my belly, I waited for the ghost of her to move again. I exhaled deeply in defeat, as I sensed she or the kicking phantom would not be returning. My mind drifted to dreaming of her instead.

In my daydream, I could see her. She was four, sitting in front of my bedroom dresser mirror as I brushed her fine, long, brown hair. Our eyes caught each other's reflection, and we would each smile in response. That preschooler then morphed into a school-aged girl who rode a bike with the wind blowing back that same dark mane, revealing a gleeful grin. Nick was there in my daydream, too, holding the wheels steady beside her as she giggled with delight down the sidewalk. Then I heard the low rumbles of clapping as a teenage girl held up a diploma. The soft strands of her straightened brown hair brushed the shoulders of her cream commencement gown. Finally, as my fantasy finished, a beautiful young woman in a white dress came into view. She was arm in arm with a silver-haired version of my husband. Opening my eyes, I watched the fan above the bed spin in silent circles. I had a vision of Nora's whole life that was supposed to be . . . but never would.

Or maybe I was given a glimpse into another dimension? A parallel universe like in *The Lion, The Witch, and The Wardrobe*, where there was a secret door that would lead me through a portal to another world—a world where she lived instead of died. I just needed to find it. I wanted to be in the universe where I got to be a mother to a living Nora. I felt foolish then for thinking back to a few days ago when I feared motherhood, its vulnerability and responsibility and all the change it would bring. Now, I would give anything to have back the chance at being her mother.

There was a knock on my bedroom door, "Lindsey, it's Mom. Can I come in?"

Over my shoulder I saw my mother poke her head through the crack of the door, like she used to do when I was a teenager. She wore a black sheath dress that ended above her knees, and the black jacket she wore to hide the short sleeves brought your attention to the pendant resting on her chest that read, "Grandma." Like me, she had little proof of her new role. Nora was her first and only grandchild, and with Nora now missing, the only thing my mother had to show for her highly-anticipated title of grandmother was a silver heart-shaped pendant she wore proudly around her neck.

With my back to her, and without moving from the fetal position I cradled myself in, I replied through sniffles, "Yes, you can."

Without saying a word, Mom slipped into bed next to me as I looked out the window at an earth buried under the weight of snow. Mom put her arm around me like she did when I was sick as a child and would sleep next to me, my spine parallel to her stomach. Her familiar perfume wafted in the air. She smelled like the fusion of roses and wine. Nora had smelled like blood and freshly-washed baby clothes. Inhaling my own mother's scent, it came to me Nora would never know mine.

Mom stroked my hair, "Hi, honey." A silent tear fell from my cheek onto the pillow at the sound of my mother's voice. Another thing Nora would miss. Uncontrollable sobs that lingered at the bottom of my throat could no longer be muffled. The ache of a cry released. Tears flowed as my body heaved. My mother held me tighter.

"I'll never get to brush her hair," I sobbed.

"I know," Mom's voice cracked back. "I know," she cried again, as she then burst into her own puddle of grief. "I won't, either."

Then I realized my pain was too much for her to hold as she moved into her own. And although I knew she was hurting and was letting me know she couldn't imagine my suffering and that's what caused hers, her comment made me think I had failed not only Nora and Nick but her, too.

Her mourning was too much for me to witness and feel because I could barely contain my own. I touched my mother's hand to comfort her. "It's okay, Mom. I'll be okay."

When there was a break in her cries, I asked her to help me get ready for the funeral. Instead of me brushing Nora's hair, my mother brushed mine. I watched her mother me from the reflection in the mirror, dropping curls from a hot iron around my face to frame it. I wondered again if I was a mother. For unlike my own mother, I had no one on whom to bestow my motherly affection.

Mom finished curling my hair into ringlets that dropped into waves upon my neck. Since Nora died before she was born, was my motherhood stillborn like Nora? I knew I was born into motherhood; my body knew this in the ache of my engorged breasts and deflated womb. I remember growing into this new person—a source of origin, Nora's beginning. But with her silent birth, my motherhood, like her life, was over before it started. Stillborn . . . failing from the start.

"All done," Mom said softly. She let the last strand of hair drop around the curve of my cheek, which accentuated the sadness in my eyes.

"Thank you, Mom." I changed out of my pajamas and into my dark mauve, long-sleeve dress. The gathered fabric in the middle hid my leftover baby bump that I unsuccessfully attempted to suck in while examining my reflected profile in the mirror. I didn't buy the dress for Nora's funeral, I had it in my closet from an autumn wedding the year before. Not wanting to wear black to my daughter's funeral, and not having the energy to face the mall, I chose the plum dress. It was the only clothing I would ever get to wear to the only event I would ever get to have for my daughter. There would never be dance recitals, graduations, or a wedding. Nora's funeral would be the only time I would ever get to be her parent in public, and I decided I would stand out by wearing dark plum, instead of blending in with the rest of the crowd dressed in black.

Opening my eyes wide in the mirror, I put the last touch of mascara on my lashes.

"You're going to wear makeup?" my mom asked with surprise.

"Yeah, I want to look my best." I broke eye contact with my reflection in the mirror to meet her reflected ones.

"Aren't you afraid it will smear when you cry?"

I shook my head. "No. I don't care if it does." I screwed my mascara brush top back onto its bottom.

"You're brave."

"It's not bravery when you have no choice," I wanted to say

back but didn't. Instead, I flashed her a small grin in the mirror before she left the room to wait for me with the others.

Opening the top dresser drawer, I pulled out a small gray box and opened it. Inside was the braided diamond ring Nick had given me on my thirtieth birthday three weeks prior, for creating and carrying Nora, for becoming a mother. The gift I was no longer sure I was entitled to.

Taking a deep breath, I carefully removed the ring from inside the box and slid it down to the base of my right-hand ring finger. Sighing, I found that it fit again. The past five days of night sweats that soaked my sheets had rid my body of all the water I had retained during the final weeks of pregnancy. I wasn't sure if the title of mother still applied to me, but to my daughter's funeral, I would wear it.

Arriving at the funeral home, Nick and I walked in holding hands with the cold winds of the dark winter night following us through the doors. Upon entering, the ugly teddy bear programs with her name and one date on them greeted us in the lobby. The funeral home's purple carpet, left from when the building was the Minnesota Vikings' corporate headquarters, created a warm cozy feeling that worked surprisingly well with the twinkling tea light candles and the aroma of pink roses that decorated each room. It was lovely, and I loathed it.

My mother had asked me a few days prior if we wanted plants at the funeral.

"No plants. I don't want to be in charge of anything else that could die."

Someone had suggested roses, and I had agreed with the caveat that they were pink roses. Not because I liked pink but because I hated it and hoped to never see a pink rose again after that night.

People had already arrived. My best friend, Staci, and our

friend Kelly, who completed our trio of three when we were teens, drove up five hours from Milwaukee on a cold January night to be there. My best friend from college, Sloane, who was my first friend I had made in the dorms, along with aunts, uncles, cousins, and my parent's friends, Nick's friends, and our coworkers attended to give us their condolences. A handful of military men who had served with Nick came dressed in their formal attire. And my eighty-year-old grandmother, never one to conform, wore an all-white, fur-lined dress and stood in front of a framed picture of Nora, sobbing familiar tears.

I tried my best to smile and nod at each person individually, giving them a silent *thank you* as I walked by, not wanting to speak to anyone. Instead, still holding Nick's hand, I led him to the one-stall bathroom and locked the door behind us.

"Dad offered to pay for the funeral," I said.

Nick fixed his silk, gold-and-blue checkered necktie that he wore with his charcoal suit, while standing in front of the bathroom sink. I didn't know anything about ties, but Nick's wasn't even crooked.

He shook his head and replied with the answer I knew he would give. "No way." And both of us knew why. This was the only time he got to be Nora's dad. The only thing he would ever get to do for his daughter was pay for her funeral.

People gathered in the simple and sparse chapel waiting for the ceremony to begin. Nick and I walked toward the front row of the pews amongst the candlelight as soft berceuse music played. Nora's ashes in her urn were up on a small altar next to a black-and-white, eight-by-ten photo of her, and a pink rose someone had placed there. I felt a small genuine smile relax upon my face as it was all stunningly beautiful . . . like her.

Our mothers on either side of us sat in the front row. One hand held my mother's, while my other hand held Nick's. At some point during the ceremony, the officiant introduced us as Nora's mom and dad, and my spine stiffened. It was the first time we were referred to by that title in public. It felt both foreign and familiar. Tonight, everyone saw us as Nora's parents, but tomorrow would they see our parenthood?

The officiant said a few words, read a prayer, and then a poem, before he asked if I or Nick wanted to say anything. I hadn't planned on it, unsure of what to say about such a short life, but I found myself letting go of my mother's and Nick's hands and moving toward the microphone. There, in that space, I got to be Nora's mother . . . if only for a moment. Opening my mouth to speak, the words I needed to say found me and fell from my lips through silent tears. I held tightly to the wooden podium to steady myself. Briefly, I looked up to see my loved ones gathered as they listened and became a sea of weeping faces blurred by my words. I focused on my breath and said whatever came to my lips, but the only elegy I would remember was, "All she knew was love."

Which was true. Nora would never know the smell of rain on freshly cut grass or see sunbeams as they broke through a clouded sky, but it also meant she would never have to know the pain of having your heart broken from losing someone you love. For nine months, Nick and I only sent her love through the veil of skin that separated her world from ours. Maybe Omar Khayyam was correct when he wrote in *The Rubaiyat*, "He who never lived a moment is happy. That man is at peace whose mother never bore him." Peace was all Nora ever knew.

After the ceremony, Nick and I stood in front of a line of our guests. We shook hands, received hugs, and thanked them for coming, just as we'd done a year and half ago at our wedding. All the same faces were here again, this time with sorrowful expressions. After the line of condolences was finished, we made our way into the lounge room for sandwiches and snacks. The ritual of satiating yourself, nourishing your life with food while mourning another body's death, seemed odd to me.

"Why do we need food at a funeral?" I asked my dad, who stood next to me against the floral wallpaper wearing a black suit jacket with a charcoal turtleneck under it.

"So people have something to do."

Overwhelmed and clouded by sorrow, I asked naively, "Death makes people hungry?"

"No," Dad scoffed with a grin. "Grief makes people uncomfortable. The food is to give them something to do so they feel less so."

Before I had a chance to respond, we were met by my uncle Andy who approached us wearing the same suit he wore to my wedding. Andy was handsome like my father, but as the younger brother, he looked older. His own grief had added years to his face.

"I'm sorry Tash couldn't make it. She's taking care of the new baby and all." He told this truth as gently as he could.

I nodded my head in acknowledgment. Andy's second daughter, my cousin Tasha, and I had shared birthday parties together at Grandma's house growing up since we both had December birth dates, hers just a year and a week behind mine. Tash and I were both excited to find out we were pregnant at the same time, due in the same month as our own birthdays, two weeks apart, and whichever baby came first would be Grandma's first great-grandchild.

Tasha's son, Quinn, was born sixteen days before Nora, on the day of the Sandy Hook massacre. I remembered receiving the news of Quinn's joyful arrival through emoji-filled texts from Grandma. I cried as I watched cherub faces of kindergarteners who had just been stolen from their parents by a mass shooter flash on the large, flat-screen television in our living room and in most living rooms across America. Hearing of one mother's birth into motherhood while another's motherhood was just taken away, I rubbed Nora through the barrier of my belly, grateful she was safe inside of me, tucked away from the dangers of this world. At the time, I was unable or unwilling to imagine then what it was like to lose a child, telling myself that happens to other people. It was a lie I let myself believe so I didn't have to get too close to another parent's unimaginable pain.

Two weeks later, I was the one in a funeral parlor. Why did Tasha get to keep her baby? Was it because she paid the gods penance around motherhood already, losing her own mother to cancer three years prior? I recalled crying into a pillow while pregnant with Nora, missing Aunt Mary and feeling sad for Tash, wondering what it had been like for her as she entered motherhood as a child without a mother. I never thought everyone would eventually be crying tears of sadness for me, the mother without a child.

"Well, you know how it feels." Mom had quietly joined our circle, filling in the silence,

Andy shook his head, "No. I don't know what it's like." I furrowed my brow toward him, momentarily confused by his response until he continued, "I've never lost a child."

When he said this, it resonated with me, but at the time I didn't know why. I simply replied, "Thank you," as he left. It wasn't until years later I would learn my uncle had taught me my first lesson in how to support the bereaved. With his simple and honest words, he honored each of our losses by acknowledging their differences.

Both are painful. Their similarity lies in the suffering grief brings, but the things we grieve are as unique as the person we lost and the role they played in our lives.

He grieved for what had been, and I grieved for what could have been. I couldn't begin to know his pain, and he didn't pretend to know mine. By being honest about these differences in grief, he held space for what both grievances have in common—suffering.

Left alone, I willed myself to be a wallflower, camouflaging sadness from others among the wall's floral print where I stood. From the corner of my eye, I saw my cousin's pregnant wife, Christina, sitting on the antique Victorian sofa in the reception room. Her stomach round and taut under her form-fitting, black, maternity dress accentuated her seven month's pregnant belly. No matter where I looked or who I talked to, I couldn't escape the cruel fact that most babies live, just not mine. I watched with curiosity as Christina dotted tissues under her eyes, crying for a baby she never met. What kind of person has the courage to go to a baby's funeral pregnant? I shook my head at my own dissociation, temporarily forgetting this had happened to me. That it sucked to be me! My cousin and his wife still had their baby; ours was dead. Diverting my eyes, I walked past Christina and her round, expecting midsection with an empty drink in hand.

By myself, I steadied my elbows against a vacant cocktail table when the sea of people around me suddenly became wavy, rhythmic, and I started to feel sick. I had lost Nick in the crowd over a half-hour before, my life raft gone, and tasting bile build in the back of my throat, I took refuge in a private office down the hall, far away from others. Slowing my breath, the seasickness subsided. Rhythmically, I rocked myself back and forth in the office's swivel chair. Through the window I watched the lights on the houses across the street twinkle, like a string of stars, leftover from Christmas.

Clutching Nora's footprint pendant that hung around my neck with the hand that wore the mother ring I didn't believe I deserved, I asked aloud, "Nora, where are you? Why couldn't you stay?" but there was no answer. Still swaying in the chair, I watched snow dance in the beams of light outside the office window and recalled the hike we had taken the day before she died. This snowfall and that snowfall reminded me of her.

About twenty minutes later, Nick found me in my hiding spot. He touched my shoulder from behind before telling me everyone had left, and it was time for us to go home, too. We grabbed our coats from the foyer before Nick held the door of the funeral home open for us to descend into the blackness of the night. I walked out the entryway carrying my baby's ashes in a tiny box that fit into one gloved hand. After today, would the world remember I was a mother? All I had to show for my motherhood was an urn with an ugly ceramic teddy bear on it.

"This isn't fair," I whispered to Nick. My words hung like white smoke against the black air.

"No, it's not," he said with his eyes on his daughter's urn between my fingers.

The darkness of our long winter ahead had just begun.

chapter 10

A MOTHER'S
INTUITION

Maybe I was warned? There were signs. The vision I had of her name on a gravestone. The feeling I would be pregnant three times, not twice like I planned. The voice on the walk in the woods when I last felt Nora truly move that said, "Remember this." Why did I shut the nursery door before I left for the hospital?

There were other warnings, too. Ones given to me years before her birth and others given recently in the weeks before she was born. They haunted me as I tried sleeping the night after her funeral. Lying in bed next to Nick passed out, his head heavy on the pillow from heartache, I watched bright, colorful, cartoon images glow from the television, illuminating the window curtains and walls. Mute DVR reruns of *Family Guy* still danced across the screen until morning. Turning toward Nick sleeping on my old side of the bed, I listened for the rhythm of inhales and exhales as he breathed. Anxious he might suddenly stop respiring in his sleep. Fearing night would continue to betray us, letting Death creep into our room again.

Watching his chest rise and fall, I remembered the first Friday of December when I had come home from work earlier than usual. On my way to the bedroom to change out of my maternity work slacks and sweater, I bumped into Nick in the hallway. He seemed shaken and disoriented, rubbing his palm into his right eye, having just woken from a nap.

"What's wrong?" I asked, as afternoon shadows from trees fell across the hallway floor. Outside all branches were bare, but the brown grass was waiting for the first snow to cover nature's floor. Winter, like our grief, had not yet arrived.

Letting the hallway wall brace his back, Nick softly said, "I had the worst dream."

"Yeah?" Mirroring his motion, I leaned against the wall. My large belly with Nora inside made it uncomfortable to stand.

"I dreamed that . . ."—he took a deep breath—"I fell asleep on the couch with Nora on my chest and when I woke up, she was"—his shoulders dropped as exhaled—"dead."

Surprised but not stirred, I wrapped my arms around him. "Oh, honey." I held him in a hug a little longer than habit, hoping to ward off his worries. "That's awful." With my wrist still resting on his neck, I pulled away, my eyes meeting his. "It's just a dream," and then kissed his clean-shaven cheek for reassurance.

"I know." He shook his head, still shaken. "But, it felt so real."

Motioning that I was moving into the bedroom, I made my way to the mattress and took a seat. Nick followed behind and leaned his back against my antique dresser. George jumped up onto the bed and settled next to me as I changed out of my work clothes and into comfy ones. "It makes sense you would have that dream." I struggled to strip off a sock from my swollen foot. "You're just worried about the responsibility of becoming a parent."

Nick seemed more settled after my answer. His hands that had tightly held the dresser behind him loosened their grip. Walking over to him, I placed one last comforting kiss on his cheek. "Here. She's moving. You can feel her." I reassured him again, positioning his palm on my basketball-sized bump. "Nora's okay."

With his hand touching my belly and his baby safely in it, he forced a smile. "You're right."

It was out of character for me to have to console my husband's worries. Just a week earlier, while sitting in my mother's hand-me-down rocking chair in Nora's nursery, it was I seeking reassurance from him. When putting away the gifts we had received at Nora's baby shower, I was plucking off the price tag of a pacifier. "What if something happens and we have to return everything?"

Nick stopped lining up newborn diapers under the changing table and stated assuredly, "Nothing is going to happen."

Rolling away from Nick while in bed, I shifted beneath the covers, being careful not to bump my bottom against his as my vagina was still swollen. Listening to the hum of the fan, I remembered the summer after Nick and I had started dating. While walking home from biology class, I noticed a yellow flier on a campus kiosk for a psychic. The psychic's address was in my neighborhood, a few blocks from where I lived off campus. I decided to stop by, wanting to know if the universe also thought Nick might be my Mr. Right.

An older woman, with taut wrinkles around her thick, black-mascaraed eyes answered the door of the small corn-colored stucco home. I held up the flier from campus and she let me in. Her over-the-shoulder shawl fluttered in the wind as she closed the door behind me. The smell of incense permeated her home. She gestured for me to sit on her oversized sofa in front of a coffee table, where she sat down next to me. Without exchanging names, she handed me a deck of tarot cards and motioned for me to shuffle. I paused to take off my backpack that blocked the breeze from the window fan I heard humming. Sweat dripped down the nape of my neck as I shuffled the cards and placed them on the worn wood.

"What questions will you ask the cards?" she asked, with a sweeping hand gesture.

I bit my lip, a little embarrassed. "I want to know if the current man I'm dating is 'the one.'"

She then laid six cards out across the scratched wood in what was called a "True Love" spread. Two cards were placed side by side above the center of the rectangular table. Then three cards were placed beneath those and finally one single card under the row of three. The top two cards she told me represented mine and my current partner's feelings for each other. "You both love each other very much." She looked away from the cards and at me once more with a knowing smile. "But you haven't told each other yet."

I nodded and blushed. Nick and I wouldn't exchange *I love yous* until later that winter.

Flipping over the next row of three rectangles, she inspected them. "*Hmmm.* Yes," rattled up from the bottom of her throat. "You and this man complement each other, yes?" Her makeup-framed eyes met with mine momentarily. "You don't *need* each other but *want* each other. This is good."

Moving to reach for the final card, she raised her eyebrows enticingly and informed me, "This is called the true love card." Holding my breath, I watched as she flipped it over and predicted, "You will marry this man."

I brought my hands up to my mouth in a satisfied silent prayer position when a breeze from the window fan blew over the top card from the deck that had been placed beside the overturned ones on the table.

"Ah, we must use this." The psychic held up the runaway card she had caught. "Fate blew it your way." She placed it next to the other six, image side facing up. "What do you want to ask this card?"

Not sure of what else I wanted to know, I asked the next logical question. "Will we have children?"

The psychic squinted as she studied the colorful card with a sun and moon celestial circle that had wolves howling toward the shape. "Yes," she said, but hesitated.

I sensed a shift in her posture. "Is something wrong? Will the baby be... healthy?" The still young and naïve before-Nora-died me thought that a health challenge would be insurmountable. The after-Nora-died me longed for a living baby. For no matter what challenge my child might face, I would still love her unconditionally. After all, I loved a dead child. Nothing seemed more challenging than that.

The psychic bobbed her head, looking only at the card and not at me. "Yes. Your baby will be healthy." I let out a held-back breath, ignoring her silent "but." I should have asked if my baby would be born alive. But I didn't because nobody ever thinks their baby is going to be born dead.

Still not able to sleep, I grabbed my phone, which now had a picture of Nora's little lifeless body with her mouth slightly ajar as the background image for both my locked and home screen. While trying to commit the lines of her heart-shaped pale face to memory, I recalled that my previous thought wasn't completely true. A part of me knew it could happen. Babies could die. Nora was not the first dead newborn I'd seen. I closed my eyes and imagined another mother's dead baby that burned into the backs of my eyelids.

In graduate school while studying abroad in India, my classmates and I would wake in our modern western hotel in Dharamsala that had running water, flushable toilets, and a view of the Tsuglagkhang Temple (the Dalai Lama Temple), where we meditated in His Holiness's presence. As a group of mostly white suburban Midwest women, we walked to class each morning down the mountainside over large boulders to a school building where we studied Tibetan medicine. One day on this dirt path, we passed an Indian woman carrying her child. The baby looked sick and malnourished. Her baby wasn't moving or crying. The baby's face was sunken, with skin tightly pulled over cheekbones and flies swarming in and out of her baby's parted lips.

I wouldn't admit to myself then that this woman's baby had died. I don't think the mother could admit it to herself, either. But now having held a lifeless child, I believe that hers, like mine, was dead. Her baby's mouth hung open, the same way Nora's did in the delivery room.

This mother walked the dusty streets that smelled of savory spices mixed with sour sweat in her sandals and a stained sari. Her baby's lifeless face protruded from the bundled, soiled sling against her breast. I saw her stop by groups of Indian men on the road begging for money, for food, for kindness. Pleading for help. But they would not help her. I did not help her.

I didn't meet the mother's gaze. I did, however, gawk at her child. I knew it was wrong, privileged even, but I did it anyway, not knowing what else to do. Since I didn't speak Hindi, I couldn't understand what the mother was saying to the men, but in her eyes that I tried hard to avoid were all the words one needed to understand. She was desperate. Desperate to have her baby back.

I am that mother. Sometimes I think I'm being punished for not helping her.

Or maybe she was a foreshadow of my own fate, like when a chimera appeared to Greek sailors before the arrival of their future misfortunes. For if someone saw her, the fire-breathing beast with a lion's face, a goat's horns, and serpent's tail—a shipwreck, a terrible storm, death, or in my case, a dead baby usually followed.

Tossing and turning in bed, I tried moving the memory out of my mind, but a more recent one took its place.

After our last doctor's appointment ten days ago, where we scheduled our induction date for Nora, I called my parents from the car on the way home to give them an update. There was a lack of cervical effacement and absent progression on dilation. The doctor had stripped my membranes one more time in hopes of moving labor along.

"Are you sure that's safe?" my mom or dad asked as they listened to me on speakerphone.

"The doctor wouldn't do it if it wasn't," I said, frustrated that my parents were already challenging my parenting choices.

Second guessing my already-made decision after the conversation with my parents, I started Google searching "membrane sweep" and "stripping membranes" once I got home. I'm not sure why I worried. I already had the procedure done once, a week earlier, and nothing had happened, so why would it cause a problem now? But lying on my side on the couch, propped up by pillows supporting Nora in my midsection, I couldn't push away the image of the doctor's blood-stained glove after she completed the sweep. Just for reassurance that I made a proper parenting decision, I clicked on the link to an internet baby forum thread and read responses to the original question of, "Did you strip membranes to induce labor?"

There were many comments that said it was helpful. One woman wrote she went into labor the next day, and another commented that within an hour after the sweep, her contractions started. Momentarily relieved, I audibly exhaled, but before I finished scrolling through the responses, I read one replier's post who wrote in all caps, "DON'T STRIP MEMBRANES. MY FRIEND'S BABY DIED."

My heart rate skyrocketed. I did my best to calm down by reminding myself my baby was fine. She was bumping against my bladder as I read the cautionary words on the screen, reminding me I needed to pee. That woman's friend's baby must have had something else wrong. Almost certain I was safe from such a fate because all the other moms on the thread swore by the sweep, I told myself losing a baby happened to other people. Besides, I couldn't go back and undo it.

I lay awake studying the picture of my beautiful but dead daughter in the black-and-white photo on my phone, uttering under my breath, "But it did happen. It happened to us."

chapter 11

IT HAPPENED
TO US

The day after her funeral, I continued my new daily ritual of making a nest on the couch. Like Linus, I dragged my favorite blanket, a down comforter, with me from room to room. I usually ended up curled under it, reading in front of the smoky fire Nick kept going for the past week to combat the cold we not only felt from the biting winter outside but from the bitter emptiness inside our bodies. Since my Google God refused to respond to my prayers, I had turned to Amazon for answers in books or what psychology refers to as bibliotherapy—using reading material for help in solving personal problems or in my case, advice about how I might survive this thing called "grief." Like the fire, I burned with needing to find other brokenhearted mothers' stories about how they had survived losing a child and even went on to have another baby.

Although I had just delivered a full-term baby one week ago, all I wanted was to be pregnant again. Well, all I wanted was for Nora to be here, even if it was just being pregnant with her again. Bringing one hand to my deflated balloon of a belly covered in silk pajamas, I wished I had cherished every moment with Nora more and never complained about being pregnant. But if I couldn't have Nora, then maybe one day I could still have another baby? Curious if other women with stillborn babies felt the same as me, I downloaded Elizabeth McCracken's memoir on the stillbirth of her first son and birth of her second, *The Exact Replica of a Figment of My Imagination.*

Settled onto the couch, I nodded my head along with every electronic page. I devoured the book in an evening and shouted, "Yes!" multiple times throughout the memoir. Each sentence she wrote was how I felt. Finishing it in front of the crackling heat of the fire's glow, I mouthed the last line of her book as I read, "It's a happy life, *and* someone is missing. It's a happy life . . ."

I desperately wanted to be happy. But I couldn't imagine finding the innocent Lindsey I used to be, who believed in good fortune and experienced laughter so easily. How could I find happiness again when someone was forever missing? C.S. Lewis, who I had also recently discovered in my search for answers, kept journals after his wife's death, *A Grief Observed,* and described grief as an amputation. No prosthetics would ever be able to replace the limb of Nora I had lost.

With my eyebrows furrowed, I shook my head. *No Elizabeth, you must be the exception. Some kind of magical unicorn that has found her way out of grief as one couldn't possibly be both bereft and content.*

Closing the cover of my Kindle in frustration, I dropped it on the coffee table where a white gift bag was stuffed with condolence cards from last night's funeral. Eyeing the bag, I debated if then was the time to open those freshly bandaged wounds. Nick sat next to me on the couch, where he took turns stroking the stubble on his chin and mouthing each word that he read from *Man's Search for Meaning.* He seemed to be searching for answers in the book he said was his favorite on our first date. Both of us were in a game of hide-and-seek with the questions death left behind. It seemed as good as time as any, to pick at our barely scabbed-over scars and run the salt of other people's tears into them.

Phases of loss fell from the inscriptions next to signatures.

"I had a miscarriage" more than one in four of the cards read. "We lost our second baby at thirteen weeks pregnant this past fall." Another card announced another member of the secret club we were being let into that we didn't know existed—a club you never wanted to be a part of for the dues were too high. "We had a four-month-old who died thirty years ago. He would be around your age now," a cursive-filled letter on ruled writing paper revealed.

The answer to my question of who had survived losing a baby was waiting for us from within the folds of the handwritten messages. Friends and family we thought we shared everything with, shared with us their secrets of children lost during pregnancy or after birth within Hallmark condolence card confessionals.

"Why doesn't anyone talk about it?" I asked Nick, while staring at the pile of pastel cards.

He didn't have an answer. No one ever told us stillbirth was a possible outcome of pregnancy, not even our doctor. Before I broke up with Google, I had searched for statistics on stillborn babies and found it happened in 1 out of 175 pregnancies in the United States. This is the equivalent of a Boeing 747 carrying a total of approximately four hundred people on board, crashing every week for a year—21,000 stillbirths annually in the United States alone.

Everyone knows that one in four pregnancies will end in miscarriage. Barbara Kingsolver wrote in *Animal Dreams,* one of my favorite books from college, "A miscarriage is a natural and common event. All told, probably more women have lost a child from this world than haven't." That's why Nick and I secretly waited to share the news we were expecting with Nora, like most new parents do, until we were past the first twelve weeks of pregnancy and into the so-called safe zone. We foolishly thought nothing could go wrong after the first trimester.

My mind drifted back to New Year's Day when we also sat in the same spot on our green suede couch in front of the fire. Our family had opened presents for the Christmas celebration we had delayed. Everyone wiped away fresh tears as I gave them their individualized gifts meant to be given to them from Nora. My mom sat on the fireplace hearth with warm, low flames fluttering behind her and reminded me that Aunt Marie, one of my mom's sisters out of her seven siblings, had two miscarriages before she was able to have my cousins.

"We didn't think she would ever be able to have babies," Mom said of her younger sister. "Aunt Marie doesn't talk about it, but she should have a child the same age as you." My mother then said something similar to Kingsolver's quote. "But she miscarried right before I got pregnant. I guess a mother always remembers what was supposed to be."

Aunt Marie would send me a card almost twice a month the first year after Nora died, sharing with me that she never forgot about those two sparks of life that once inhabited her womb. "Who would they have been?" she wrote in one of her many notes.

Kristi had sat next to me on the couch, knees tucked under her, straightening her magenta-rimmed glasses. "And you remember how Grandma and Grandpa would always talk about Patrick?"

While I was growing up, my grandparents bantered back and forth in their 1970s-style living room to see who could make the other laugh the loudest. He would chuckle as his big belly rolled at her playful pokes, and she would shriek with her head thrown back at his inappropriate humor. Every Sunday, the whole family gathered at our grandparents' house for their burned pot roast dinners. All of us nine grandchildren would avoid eating their cooking but ate up their stories instead.

There was one story, however, where in place of the usual grin she wore, Grandma's face would become stoic, and laughter abandoned her lips. Her gaze looked past our tiny shoulders as if she was searching for someone there. It was the story of her fourth son, Patrick, who, like Nora, was stillborn.

More than halfway through her pregnancy, Grandma told her doctors she could no longer feel her baby move. "A miscarriage" they called it then, but Grandma could clearly recount the image of Patrick's little lifeless body being placed on the stainless-steel table next to her with his back to her.

"He looked like a doll I used to love when I was a little girl."

She never saw his face. She never held him. She was never given the chance. Instead, in the 1960s, they asked if you wanted to hold someone else's living baby. Grandma didn't. She sometimes forgets what year or what season he was born. She doesn't even know where he was buried. But his name was known, and his story often told between others when a memory would drift to him. I knew at a young age that I had an uncle named Patrick, who, like Peter Pan, would never grow up. There was a reason that Grandma's tears, the ones that dotted her white fur-lined dress at Nora's funeral looked so familiar. Grandma was also a bereaved mother.

"I forgot about that," I told Kristi as the fire popped. "I remember they both talked about Patrick. I guess I didn't really understand the depth of that story until now." What I meant was the depth of Grandma's pain.

My mind moved to the last memory I had of my grandfather before he was cremated almost six years prior. Cumulative grief bubbled inside of me. Grandpa was the first dead person I ever kissed. His forehead, like Nora's, was like ice against my lips.

Mom broke my memory. "I don't know if I ever told you, but remember Great-Gram, Grandma Norine, who Nora and I are named after?" Mom gulped back tears before she continued. "Her first baby—the baby born before my dad—died, too."

Great-Gram, or Gram to us, was my mother's grandmother and was the first dead person I ever saw. At age fifteen, I went to her funeral, where Gram, ninety-two when she died, looked the same dead in her casket as she did alive.

"Her baby died after he was born. I don't know if he lived for a couple of hours or a couple of days. He's buried, but no one knows his name to find his grave." Mom's voice cracked with her previous words. How sad that the baby's name was never known.

"Your grandpa, my dad, was the baby born after. I'm not sure Gram and Great-Grandpa would have had him if the other baby had lived because they had Dad soon after their first baby died."

My mom played with her new heart-shaped Nora necklace between her fingers. She was telling me I might not be alive if a baby hadn't died somewhere back in my family tree. Did Nora die because I named her after my great-grandmother, setting into destiny Nora and I to experience her same fate? A Rumpelstiltskin repayment. Our family needed to sacrifice a baby every other generation as an atonement for our opportunity to live. I shuddered, feeling saliva in my mouth thicken, like I might vomit.

Later that same day, I was still cocooned on the couch and surrounded by cards when dad called to tell us they had made it back home to southern Wisconsin safely. "Your mom and I donated money to cover a stay at Faith's Lodge," Dad said through the phone. "I think you guys should go." The grief retreat I had pooh-poohed in the hospital the day after Nora died, he had paid for in full.

I told Nick of Dad's suggestion. He reached for his laptop and searched for Faith's Lodge in his browser while he ran his right hand through Georgie's fur, who was snuggled up next to him into a curled-up, fuzzy caterpillar position on the arm of the couch.

Georgie's caterpillar shape reminded me we had prepared to be transformed into beautiful parental butterflies. However, we were turned into Virginia Woolf's moth, in her poem, "The Death of a Moth," who were dreary, depressingly colored, and mournful creatures with little chance against death, having been burned in the flame we were drawn to.

"They have a specific weekend for pregnancy and infant loss coming up in two weeks," Nick said. He nuzzled his feet under my Linus blanket and into my nest on the couch, an empty nest, one that should be filled with Nora.

"Should we go?"

chapter 12

GOD NEEDED ANOTHER ANGEL. BULLSHIT.

"This seems stupid. Why do I want to go feel bad with a bunch of other people who feel bad?" I asked Nick, as I fiddled with the heater in the car, my teeth clacking against the cold. Pouting, I wrapped myself in the orange emergency blanket Nick got out from the trunk for me at our last gas station stop to combat my complaining.

"It said on the website it's not faith-based, right?" I asked.

Nick focused on the road.

"Because I don't want to talk about how, 'God apparently has a plan,' or that bullshit saying, 'God needed another angel in heaven.'"

These were some of the well-meaning things people had said to us in our grief, but "the road to *hell* is paved with good intentions."

I continued, "Because if God was real, God would know the only arms Nora should be in are ours."

For the first ten years of my life, my sister and I were raised as Christmas and Easter Catholics, the ones who only showed up for the big holidays. It wasn't until my dad got sober and went through Alcoholics Anonymous that we all found God, my parents again, and my sister and I for the first time. From then on, I went to CCD (Confraternity of Christian Doctrine) every Wednesday after school for two hours to learn about Jesus, but mostly I just hung out with friends watching older kids sneak a smoke behind the building. Then, when I was twelve and after I took Communion, I would lie awake at night, terrified of living forever in heaven. The idea of never having an end to life was more unsettling to me than never-ending nothingness.

At seventeen, I remember going through the confirmation process, which included confession. In the late nineties, our church no longer used the confessional box, and I found myself sitting knees to knees with the priest in his long white robe while I confessed my weekly sins. I would say I wasn't nice to my sister or that I had heavy-petted with my high school boyfriend over the weekend. I really didn't care what I said, as I didn't want to get confirmed, because I didn't believe in the God I grew up with.

I told my mom this in the kitchen of my childhood home, between the country wooden dining room table and our new portable phone with caller ID and call-waiting. "I don't want to get confirmed!" I said passionately, in my annoyed seventeen-year-old tone.

"You don't want to become a soldier of God?"

My eyes rolled so far into the back of my head, I didn't see her reaction when I huffed, "I don't believe in God!"

Though, I heard very clearly what she said next. "If you don't get confirmed, I'll take away your car."

Arms crossed, and a hip pushed out to one side, I squinted, held her gaze, and shouted, "I don't think it's supposed to work that way!"

I was confirmed the next Sunday. I really liked my car.

GOD NEEDED ANOTHER ANGEL. BULLSHIT.

◢◢◢

Two hours later, Nick and I pulled up in front of Faith's Lodge and parked underneath its awning. The building was three stories high with a layer of white snow upon its many roofs. Stone and redwood siding framed its picture windows. Set against the backdrop of a pine and birch-wooded forest, the lodge nestled next to a small frozen pond, large enough to go canoeing in the warmer months. By the entrance hung a sign with a green leaf that had a profile silhouette cutout of a young girl with a ponytail in its center. To my surprise, the place was more beautiful than in the photos from the brochure we received at the hospital.

Inside, we met Liz, a fifty-something female staff member, who put on her winter boots to help us unload our suitcases from our vehicle, along with the new executive director, Kelly, a forty-year-old, spunky, business professional dressed in a chunky white wool sweater. We learned Kelly was a bereaved aunt who took the position after her school-aged nephew died in a freak accident on the playground. Kelly and Liz greeted us with good, old-fashioned, Midwest nice, the kind that plowed the quarter of a mile driveway to a sad retreat center to take care of us in our sorrow.

Faith's Lodge was built in honor of a little girl named Faith who was stillborn to Mark and Susan Lacek. They created the lodge as a place they wished would have existed after the death of their first child. The silhouette profile in the leaf on the front of the building represented her. My muscles relaxed as we learned faith—the part of religion—would not be preached at the retreat.

Liz took off her tall winter boots and took us on a tour of the building. A stone gas fireplace burned in the great room that had oak-lined high ceilings and walls. In it were large caramel leather couches to sink into, with soft throws and squishy pillows. The smell of cinnamon-scented candles lingered in the air. From the dining room, there was a view of the pond, and the room had another beautiful stone fireplace, which warmed the attached kitchen. To end our tour, our host brought us to a large entryway with a big, round, wooden oak table that had an antler chandelier above it.

On the table there was a photo album with a picture on the cover of a beautiful, chubby-cheeked baby girl with a pink headband swimming in a sea of tubes and wires. A monitor was mounted on her foot that glowed red in the photo, with a hospital bracelet encircling her ankle. Her mother's arm was gently placed upon the wide-eyed baby girl's back, holding her up into a sitting position to take the photo, as she floated among the coils of plastic keeping her alive.

"This is where you can put a picture of your child if you like," Liz explained.

Nick and I nodded in silent agreement. My chest tightened as my heart ached with the understanding that this very pink, very alive baby girl was also dead. I tried imagining the pain one must have of losing a child you've locked eyes with, but the pressure of the thought hurt so much my mind could not fully comprehend the sorrow.

What was it like to watch your child die? To watch them suffer as they struggled to live? I liked to think Nora never suffered, but I really didn't know. My only hope was that Nora slipped silently away, out of consciousness and free of earthly anguish.

"You'll be staying in Kaitlin's Suite. It's up the stairs and on the left," said Liz, pointing to the large staircase that ended in front of the circular oak table. "Dinner will be ready in an hour."

We thanked her for her kindness and then headed up to our room to unpack. I wanted to hide . . . get out of my sweater and leggings and into the baggy pajamas I had been accustomed to at home for the last three weeks. The elastic in my pants pushed against and revealed my dwindling dead-baby bump. But it didn't make sense to change before dinner, so I immersed myself in the book I had brought, *The Happiness Project* by Gretchen Rubin.

I had put the book on the backburner before Nora died, since I had been busy perusing pregnancy magazines and reading weekly growth updates on my BabyCenter app. I was already joyful and didn't need a book to teach me how to be any more so. But since I had fallen out of happiness (to put it very lightly), I thought I could use some tips on how to get unstuck from this sorrow. Also, I hoped I may be able to hurry the whole Elisabeth Kübler-Ross-five-stages-of-grief thing along by focusing on cheerful thoughts instead of sad ones. I feared I might get trapped in my mourning if I dwelled too long in its house.

I decided reading a memoir about how to project your way to happiness would be the farthest thing away from dead-baby grief and might provide me with a road map back to the elusive happiness Elizabeth McCracken claimed she had found after her son died. Maybe I could even project my way through grief the way Rubin projected her way to contentment?

Nick interrupted my reading as I lay on the bed with a birch wood frame. He encouraged me to come downstairs for dinner. I didn't want to. I could have hidden in the comfy room with our own gas fireplace and view of the little lake for the whole weekend. However, I realized I was becoming selfish in my mourning. Going down to dinner with him was a small gesture of acknowledging his way of grieving and to support his needs and not only mine. I grabbed Nora's white-framed photo.

When we reached the landing at the end of the staircase, the table that once held just one baby's picture now held three more. There was a framed photo of a doll-sized little boy wearing a blue hat with his hand gently pressed against his face. It looked like he had fallen asleep sucking on his thumb. Then my eyes moved toward the two separate black-and-white photos in their own frames, one of a beautiful boy's feet and another of a gorgeous girl wearing a tiny knit hat. Both babies, with translucent skin, could have fit in the palm of a hand. Bringing my fingers to my lips, I placed a kiss onto them and then onto Nora's in the frame. I put her picture down on the table with the other forever babies and headed to dinner.

Over a salty, homemade, ground beef-and-green-bean-tater-tot dish covered in cheese, we all gathered around a wooden, family-style table. We ate quietly at first, as even bereaved parents didn't know what to say to comfort our fellow bereaved because no words really bring us much consolation.

It was the petite, friendly, and surprisingly bubbly bereaved mom Claire, with her blond bob parted down the middle and a gray turtleneck sweater and jeans, who was the first to break the awkward silence.

"Can you tell us about your baby?" she asked the couple sitting across from her.

And that was how, like a waterfall, we all shared our stories of sadness among a cascade of tears.

The tall man with glasses was married to the shorter woman with tightly-curled brunette hair. Steve and Bethany were Gracia's parents, the chubby-cheeked baby girl I had seen in the first photo on the oak table. Gracia's parents explained 1 in 100 children were born with a heart defect in the United States, and that 100,000 of those babies born worldwide with a heart defect would sadly not reach their first birthday. Gracia had died the previous October, having lived eighty-two days never leaving the hospital.

Ylonka, seated at the head of the table, introduced herself as Mateo's mom. Single with long, dark hair and an East Coast accent from New Jersey, she lost her only child due to uterine rupture from medical negligence when she was twenty-seven weeks pregnant. Like so many other women of color, Ylonka, an Afro-Latinx mother, and her son, Mateo, were victims of a healthcare system steeped in white supremacy. Ylonka shared with us the appalling reality that women of color have significantly higher rates of pregnancy loss, stillbirth, and infant death than white women. Mateo, the boy who looked like he was sucking his thumb in the photo, had died soon after he was born.

College sweethearts, Taylor and John, were Charlie's parents. Taylor was petite and blond with a warm welcoming smile, while John had broad shoulders, bushy, black hair and an actor's grin. Charlie was the couple's second child and first son, who was born at nineteen weeks the previous July due to preterm labor. One in nine babies in the United States are born prematurely. Charlie lived for five minutes.

Claire, the bubbly woman who started the conversation, introduced herself as Abigaile's mom. She and her more reserved husband, Lincoln, delivered their third child early also because of preterm labor. Abigaile was born around Thanksgiving when Claire was twenty-three weeks pregnant. Abigaile died later that day.

I admit, I was secretly jealous of Abigaile and Charlie's parents because they had older children. Did having other little hands to hold make their grief easier? They still got to be parents in the way Nick and I wanted so badly to be. But then again, maybe their other children reminded them of what they were missing. We didn't know what it was like to have a child past their due date. Was it both a curse and a blessing?

Nick and I also shared about Nora. Tears rained down our cheeks as we relayed the trauma of the day she died and was born.

With every child's story told, the other grieving parents in the room nodded along, like bobblehead dolls. The others' stories of sadness reflected their own.

"And you're never really safe," Lincoln said, placing a fork on his finished plate. "Have you read the journals where you can share your child's story?"

We all had at least seen them on the side tables or desks in our bedrooms. The journals were filled with stories of the short lives children had lived, written by bereaved parents who had stayed at the lodge. Every guest left a piece of their child's memory behind in the diaries tucked into nightstands, hoping to provide comfort to other bereft parents and let them know they were not alone in their sorrow.

I read every story in the leather-bound journal in Kaitlin's room. The diary held photos of infants who never left NICU bassinets, pictures like Nora's of babies born still, a second-grade school photo of a little boy who would never show up for picture day the following year, a teenager's senior photo who never made it to graduation, and a family portrait of a young toddler on her mother's lap that would remain empty during their next family photo shoot. Every picture in the journal was a snapshot of a happier occasion in the life of a child who was now forever missing from future photos.

Learning about all the ways your living children or future children could die was terrifying. It's part of the collateral damage that comes with finding support in other grieving parents' experiences. You find comfort in knowing you're not the only one who walks this lonely road of despair, but you also find out there is nothing extraordinary about the nature of death. You learn death likes to hide in plain sight. It's the ordinary, small everyday things that steal children from their parents.

At one point, later in my mourning, I even made a list of all the ordinary everyday things that could kill a child: pieces of raw carrots and apple slices cut too big; hot dogs and grapes not sliced four ways; pools left uncovered; backs turned to bath tubs; bacteria; misplaced or missing chromosomes; the flu; minute malignant cells; car seats improperly installed; bee stings; peanut butter sandwiches; shellfish; blankets and pillows; school shooters; drunk drivers; texting while driving; and sleep. Sleep scared me the most. For it was in my own slumber where Death stole Nora in the night.

"How does that quote go? Having children is like going around wearing your heart on the outside of your body," Ylonka said with a sigh that signaled a sense of surrender.

"Why doesn't anyone warn you?" Lincoln addressed all of us as we sat in a circle.

"Would we have listened?" Taylor asked.

She was right. None of us wanted to think about Death, possibly fearing we could invoke her with our thoughts alone, knowing she lurked in the corners of everyday life. It's easier to deny Death, especially when you're enjoying gestating with new life. Death was supposed to come at the end of life. Not before it had even begun.

Since everyone was farther from their loss than Nick and I were, I asked what had been meddling in my mind. "How do you do it? How do you carry the weight of the grief around with you each day?"

They all mostly answered, "With God."

Having matured since childhood, I made sure not to roll my eyes this time and respected other people's beliefs.

"But I imagine you prayed to God when you were about to lose your child? How do you believe in God when God didn't answer your prayers?" My brow lowered as I pushed back against faith.

Claire, a devoted Christian, answered, "He answered many of my prayers before. He simply said, 'Not this time,' to this one."

Not this time? My eyes widened at her response, but I clamped my mouth shut. It's kind of an important time to intervene. *If not now, when is the right time to phone in a favor?* I kept my commentary to myself.

The rest of the weekend was spent painting birdhouses and heart-shaped rocks in memory of our children and sharing their stories.

We made fun of how macabre it was to be on a retreat for sad parents with dead babies, knowing it's exactly where we needed to be. We ate and played board games; we laughed with guilt for laughing when our children never would. We talked about music, marathons, sports teams, jobs, and our dead children like it was a perfectly normal thing to do and not a conversation killer. Nick and I had been warned speaking about Nora could ruin a discussion. But there, in that place, with those people, it was woven within it, like the quilt of comfort the lodge wrapped us in.

chapter 13

GOD'S PLAN
SUCKS

There is a ritual at Faith's Lodge to leave behind a heart-shaped rock with your child's name on it among the other stones placed in honor of children who had left this earth too soon. We learned heart stones appeared naturally in nature and were not difficult to find on any beach. Our rocks came from the clear blue shores of Lake Superior, where Nick and I planned to spread Nora's ashes when the warmer months arrived.

The last morning at the lodge, Nick and I hiked down to the frozen pond, hand in hand, to find a spot to place Nora's stone, which we had painted yellow with her name written in white.

Walking the trail other bereaved parents had taken before us, we stopped to read the quotes burned into plywood signs and nailed into the sharp-scented pine trees that lined the path.

"Promise me that you'll always remember you're braver than you believe, stronger than you seem, and smarter than you think," A. A. Milne's Christopher Robin said to Pooh.

I wasn't moved by Christopher Robin's words. I didn't feel brave; I felt broken and angry at my body for not saving my baby. "Strong" was out of the question, and no matter how smart I was, I felt unable to make sense of the world ever since Nora died.

But maybe, it was Christopher Robin's words that inspired me to summon up the courage to ask Nick a question that had been on my mind. "Do you think we are being punished because we don't believe in God?" I shivered underneath my winter jacket and thick, wool scarf.

Nick stayed silent as we continued to walk on the winter-covered trail within the forest before he answered, "If there was a God, I don't think that's how God would work." His gloved hand squeezed my mitten one. "Besides, why would God take away our new friends' babies, too? They believed, and their babies still died."

He had a point. But wouldn't the answer be because God had a plan? Curious, I asked, "Do you believe in God now?"

"I'm not sure what I believe anymore."

I nodded my head in agreement. After what happened to us, it seemed fair that the most likely answer was to not know the answer.

Ducking under a branch, he continued, "But no, I really haven't changed my stance. I don't know if or what there is. I just know that I don't know, and that I don't believe in the faith I grew up with. It's appealing to think that God exists and believe that we might someday see Nora again, but I don't think it's true." Nick's exhale rose like a cloud in the cold air. For a moment we were quiet. The swish of our arms brushed against the sides of our puffer coats like a beat against the breeze. We walked under the naked branches of the trees contemplating the cosmos.

"Do you think it would be easier if we did believe in God?" Curious for a different perspective, I wondered if he thought that having faith might have taken the edge off some of our pain.

Nick shrugged his shoulders. "Maybe. Maybe not. That would mean God took away Nora for some higher purpose. You know, part of God's plan." The inflection in his voice became briefly sarcastic, "And 'everything happens for a reason.' But, if there is a God, I don't think God has a plan or a reason."

"I think it would be harder if we did believe," I said, taking in nature's beauty of tall pine trees covered in white, a cold clear blue sky filled with marshmallow clouds above, and the sounds of creation surrounding us. "I would just be angry with God."

"Yes, that's what I mean," he said, without looking up from the footprints he was leaving in the snow.

"What do you believe, then?" I asked.

"I'm not sure I understand your question."

"Like, do you believe in spirits?" I blushed, uneasy at the admittance of the idea.

Nick, a slight step ahead of me, stopped for a second and smirked over his shoulder. He shook his knit hat-covered head. "No."

"What about energy?" I hoped Nick thought my cheeks were red from the cold and not from embarrassment.

Walking in step with each other again and interlocking gloved hands, I noticed his forehead wrinkled with one skeptical eyebrow lifted. "Huh?"

Taking a deep breath, I summoned some courage to answer as best as I could. "I read this blog post from NPR called 'Planning Ahead Can Make a Difference in the End,' where Aaron Freeman writes that you want a physicist to speak at your funeral because, from a physics perspective, we're all energy, and according to the second law of thermodynamics, energy in the universe does not get created or destroyed. And understanding this idea of conservation of energy could help the grieving, since energy does not die. Therefore in some way, we don't die because we're all energy. Once we pass away, 'We're just less orderly,' the physicist says."

In response to my idea of atoms that live on in a forever afterlife Nick responded, "Maybe, I'm not sure," and shrugged again.

He was consistent in his response. Nick was consistent at being consistent, which I loved about him.

Approaching the pond, I stopped asking Nick about the afterlife, understanding this might be where we would deviate slightly in our grief. For me, ever since Nora died, I felt more connected to everything on earth, like there was another layer to the cosmos I had been missing until she departed. The reason the idea of energy resonated with me was because I could still feel her. Ever since I woke up at the hospital on the day after she died, I knew she was gone, but at the same time, it *felt* like she was there.

When I was pregnant with Nora, I never talked to her out loud through the veil of skin that separated yet connected us between our two worlds. Our conversation took place in my mind. And the conversation didn't stop once she died. I never really knew her outside of me, so maybe there was a made-up place in my head where she still resided. But even in her death, I still sensed something true of her in me.

By the bank of the frozen water, not far from the trail, we found an old dead oak tree with snow in the wrinkles of its bark. The trunk of the tree stood over six feet tall with sharp edges on top where it had been broken in half—the upper part missing. The inside of the remaining stump was cracked and hollowed, left empty and exposed to the harsh elements of a cruel Mother Nature. It looked like how I felt—used up, broken, and beaten down by the storm of heartbreak. It was exactly where I wanted Nora's stone to be, inside something that was beautifully broken, like me. Like her.

My mittened hand was still interlaced with Nick's as I brought the other one holding Nora's rock close to my face and whispered, "Goodbye, Nora. I will always love you." Kissing the smooth stone, it was cold, like her skin was, against my lips.

Silently, I then handed Nora's heart stone to Nick, who kissed it gently as he would have her forehead. I know this because he kissed me every morning in this same way. "I love you, my baby girl," he said, placing the stone on the stump of the beautifully broken tree. I ran my fingers under my eyes to catch their tears as a crisp wind washed over my cheeks.

For a moment, it felt like Nora was in the bitter breeze that blew between the tree's bare branches. I noticed black birds flying overhead, like a message sent from her to me. Logically, I knew this sounded silly. I didn't believe in God, but I believed in signs sent from the dead and that they lived on in atoms. And yet, it's just how it *felt*. It was like she was everywhere and nowhere at the same time. I felt close to her in nature . . . or maybe it had something to do with the lodge? In this place, with these people, I could be her mom, mothering her. Fellow bereaved parents knew me and referred to me as "Nora's mom." It was a kind of motherhood I never wanted and never would have chosen, but I would take whatever little taste of motherhood I could get.

Returning to our room, we readied our suitcase to leave. While we had learned we were not alone in our grief, we learned we were never safe in life from death, either. We got to experience being Nora's parents, but upon leaving, it felt like she was being taken away from us again. Outside of these walls, our parenthood would become invisible once more.

I searched for my Nora ring that I had placed in the inside zip pocket of my purse before our hike. Opening the zipper, I reached in and next to the ring in the bottom of the pouch the tips of my fingers found a pen with a tiny ribbon around it. Pulling it out, I couldn't believe what I saw. It wasn't a pen. It was the positive pregnancy test that had told me I was pregnant with Nora, which I'd shown Nick in our one-bedroom condo. I must have put it in there during the move and forgotten about it. I stared at the pregnancy test in the same way I stared at it ten months ago, with disbelief. I wasn't sure if I should laugh or cry. Was it a cruel joke from the universe, reminding me I was supposed to be happy with a baby but wasn't, or was it a sign from Nora that she was still with me somehow?

chapter 14

GRIEF
THERAPY

The numbness and bitterness of early grief had turned to sorrow. After coming home from Faith's Lodge, in the month or more after we got back, it seemed all I could do was cry. I would find myself at night lying on the floor of her nursery next to her forever-empty crib crying. I cried in the tub as warm water washed over my wiggly remains of a baby bump. My hands placed above and below my belly button searched for her in my tomb of a womb as hot tears made crescent moons on both sides of my face. Nick would find me and hold my cheek against his chest, my body still naked and submerged in the lavender-scented water as I sobbed. I cried in the car, my head hung upon the steering wheel with sad music blaring over the speakers. I cried in the shower with my knees curled up to my chest, as the beads of water rolled off my back and ran down my spine, tears and droplets meeting as they both bounced off my thighs. I cried myself to sleep on top of wet pillowcases and when I woke up, I cried some more. I cried when Nick cried and sometimes when he cried, I had no more tears to cry, so I watched him cry. Stunned and washed out, there were no more tears to give.

Mid-January, we started therapy and I cried there, too. Nick had suggested we go. Even though I was a therapist, I was not motivated to find a therapist, set up an appointment, and then go to multiple first sessions with different ones, trying to find a therapist who was a good fit. But we got lucky, and our first therapy session would lead to a long and lasting three-year relationship.

Her name was Anna, and she specialized in pregnancy loss and infant death (real happy stuff). She had fair skin and long, red hair like me, except her hair was thicker and a darker red, like orphan Annie's. It stood out against her fashionable cream sweater dress and white leggings. Anna's big green eyes accentuated her delicate, ageless features, but she was in her midthirties, about five years my senior, and like me, she was a licensed clinical social worker.

Unlike me, she had two living children who were in the family photo, along with her husband, on the desk in the corner of the office. The room, filled with house plants, had once been the living room in the 1900s-style home before it was divided as office space. Warm light came in through the floor-to-ceiling boxed windows despite icicles accumulating on the outside sills. Our new therapist sat with her back to the old empty fireplace, like Cinderella on her hearth, but Anna would end up being my fairy godmother. Nick and I faced her seated on a gray, two-cushion couch.

Nervously, I raked the rocks in the tiny sand tray on the side table next to me. Even though I practiced therapy, I was much more comfortable sitting across from the client couch than on it. There was control in that chair. You were trained to guide what happened in the session when you sat across from the client couch. For a novice therapist, it could seem scary at first, but after a while, sinking into the role was like sinking into the cushions. I wished I was in her wingback, beige chair and not on the couch for parents with dead children.

✔ ✔ ✔

The first time I went to therapy, I was seventeen and had just broken up with my high school boyfriend. We were in love for almost a year and then one day, I was the only one in love. I ended up sitting on a different couch in a middle-aged man's office in a strip mall across the street from a Dairy Queen that closed during the winter months. I found it hard to relate to the fifty-something gray-haired Sigmund Freud look-alike and only went to two sessions.

Fast forward almost ten years, where I was a college graduate with no direction in life except for my irrational fear I had somehow contracted HIV from engaging in sexual activities—not even having sex—with a handful of partners. Health anxiety had scared me into a depressed state. I spent nights awake with worry on my sister Kristi's college bedroom floor in a sleeping bag, which confirmed I once again needed therapy.

Unfortunately, it took a while to find the right therapist. The first one awkwardly placed his folding chair in front of the middle of the couch and behind a measured piece of tape approximately six feet away from where I sat. I had to yell across the room for him to hear me.

The next therapist was twenty minutes late, with her hair still wet from showering. My twenty-something, snotty self thought if I could shower and arrive on time for a morning appointment with dry hair as a non-morning person, I must be in better shape than the damp-haired, running-late therapist. Later, being a therapist that sometimes ran late, I learned therapists are flawed like all humans.

Finally, I found a wise elderly therapist who was a licensed clinical social worker. She introduced me to mindfulness techniques, Buddhist books, and ways for me to tame my overactive monkey mind, which she called my anxious thoughts. We only had a few sessions in an office like the one Nick and I currently sat in with Anna, but finding my grandmotherly therapist was another reason I became one. A degree in social work meant I could be a psychotherapist. After I stopped going to therapy, I went to graduate school to get a master's degree in social work, which was another two years of intense self-reflection.

In our first session with Anna, I was terrified. Having heard the rumor that couples who lose a child go on to lose their marriage, too, I feared that going to counseling with Nick would lead to some scary secret coming out about our marriage that I didn't know—like Nick had fallen out of love with me and into love with someone else. Perhaps he thought therapy was the right time to tell me he wanted a divorce, since the whole baby thing didn't work out.

Instead, Nick held my hand as we sat next to each other and took turns retelling the story of Nora's death. Anna nodded her head dutifully from her therapist chair as she listened to us share about our baby between sobs. The session lasted longer than the normal hour, but Anna provided us with all the time we needed without charging us for the extra thirty minutes.

Rolling a tissue between my fingers, I ended our recount of losing Nora with the only analogy that came to mind. "I feel like I ran a marathon and even crossed the finish line. Then when I was supposed to get my medal, which was a baby, they gave me a dead one instead. And even that shell of a newborn was taken away. Nine months of hard work—" I sighed as my head fell into my hands, "for nothing."

Anna's eyebrows drew together as she listened with genuine concern. She was a good therapist.

Nick and I shared our experience at Faith's Lodge—how it was wonderful and terribly sad all at the same time. I brought up

Steve and Bethany from the retreat. "I don't understand how I can miss someone so much that I didn't even know? There was a couple at the lodge who lost their two-month-old daughter, Gracia. They knew their baby; we just mourn the idea of ours," I said, palms up, conveying a sense of ambivalence I desperately hoped to have. "We didn't actually know Nora."

"But you did know her," Anna said, with such sincerity I almost believed her. "You knew the way she moved. The foods she liked that you ate. She knew the sound of your voice." Anna broke her steady gaze at me to look at Nick. "Both of your voices." Fresh tears nestled in the corners of Nick's eyes.

On the edge of her seat with her elbow on her knees, Anna leaned in, maintaining her unwavering gaze with us both and said with certainty, "Nora knew you."

I raised an eyebrow in reply to Anna's unlikely statement. "How could a baby know anything about us?"

"We know that a baby in the womb responds to sounds around the twenty-fourth week of pregnancy."

My vision blurred with hot wetness, and I bit the inside of my lip.

"Nora had many weeks of getting to know your voice. What you both sound like. The loving way in which you talked to each other." Anna nodded toward our held hands between us on the sofa. "The way you talked to her."

I would later learn hearing is one of the first senses we use to connect to the world outside the womb and one of the last senses to go when death arrives. Which meant Nora could hear us. She knew us, even from within me.

Anna slipped a subtle look at the clock on her desk before asking us what we hoped to get out of coming to therapy with her.

I surprised myself with my reply. "I don't want to be stuck in my grief. There were parents at the lodge who are farther out from their loss than us and they are still grieving. *Hard.* I don't want to be like that. Still hanging on."

Anna squinted her eyes and gave a therapist, *"Hmmm,"* as if she was saying without saying, grief wasn't something you could rush your way through. But I thought maybe I would be more immune to grief's grasp because if anyone should have enough coping skills to progress through this "new normal," it should be me, a therapist. I wanted to ask Anna what her squint meant. I'd given plenty of those ambiguous yet acknowledging looks myself to clients.

But Anna stood. Time was up, and I didn't get the chance to ask.

chapter 15

BABY LOSS
BLOGGING

In between crying and going to therapy, I started writing, and Nick started running. He prepared to run the Twin Cities Marathon taking place in October, and in the time I still had off before going back to work, I began a blog.

The blog was part of chapter five in Gretchen Rubin's book, *The Happiness Project*. I decided to try to project my way through grief like Rubin projected her way to happiness. I called it my Grief Project. I didn't think anyone would want to read a blog about dead-baby grief, but I soon found many bereaved moms start dead-baby blogs—it's a thing.

When I opened Blogger to create my new online journal, I found a blog I had started when I was nine-weeks pregnant with Nora. I had totally forgotten my short-lived dream of becoming a famous writer like Glennon Doyle, once blogger and now world-renowned author. The name of my hoped-to-one-day-be-famous blog was—and I am not kidding you—*Anxiety Girl Gets Pregnant*. I never wrote one post.

I shook my head as I stared into the screen of my laptop, searching hard for the girl who wrote that stupid title. In my next pregnancy, I would be staring down the barrel of an anxiety bullet-filled gun.

If I could even get pregnant again. Secondary infertility was another gut punch Mother Nature threw at loss moms.

I had not moved forward with my original blog because I was nervous about what clients would think if they found my anxiety-riddled ramblings online. "How is this lady going to help me when she can't even get her own amygdala in check?"

But now, my fingers floated over the keys outlining my new blog, and I no longer cared. A side effect of grief seemed to be indifference. Later in my mourning, a fellow-loss mom shared her theory that grieving moms came to the stage of "give no fucks" before most other women did. This stage of life usually happened to many women around their late thirties or early forties, when we finally stop letting movies, music, magazines, models, and males define our lives. We define our lives ourselves. At age thirty, I was officially in the "give no fucks" stage of grief and womanhood.

The premise of my Grief Project came to life on the computer screen in my lap as I sat crisscrossed in my leggings and oversized sweater on the couch. I picked one healing technique a month to apply to my grief so I could actively participate in my mourning. I mimicked my schedule after Rubin's:

The Grief Project Month by Month

January - Writing for Healing
February - Blogging Through Grief
March - Finding Friends in Grief
April - Sitting with Grief
May - Other People's Grief
June - Taking a Break from Grief
July - Remembering with Rituals
August - Reading Spiritual Books
September - Acts of Kindness to Heal

October - Healing through the Arts
November - Gratitude and Grief
December - Resting, Remembering, and Reflecting

I planned the project throughout the year, hoping it would offer a distraction over the next months of mourning, when Nick and I waited the suggested six months before we tried to conceive again.

One of my first posts on my new dead-baby blog included Grief Commandments like Rubin did with her Happiness Commandments at the beginning of her book. Here is what I wrote:

Grief Commandments

1. The pain is great because the love is great.
2. Sadness and happiness can both live within grief.
3. Just because I'm grieving doesn't mean I need to hide my joy and laughter.
4. I will not grieve alone; I need others to help me heal.
5. Nurturing myself emotionally, physically, and spiritually is healing.
6. The life of my baby has been swallowed by death, but I am not dead. Grief will not consume me.
7. My process is just that. Mine. I cannot compare it to others.
8. I will dedicate my joy and hope to my baby through a life well lived.
9. My pain is a part of me. I need to accept it in order to release it.
10. I move forward through my grief each day. It is always there, but each day it gets better.
11. I will be intentional about my grief. My grief does not control me. I control it.

Watching words become sentences on the screen, I thought my Grief Project might be a weird control-freak thing to do. I had trouble believing I would ever live up to my Grief Commandment ideals. They fell into the category of "easier said than done." Maybe even wishful thinking of how I imagined a therapist should grieve. But I was determined to see this new plan through. Maybe I could project my way through grief like it was a graduate school thesis. If I just completed all the requirements in the rubric, I might be able to map my way out of mourning and expeditiously move myself through the icky emotions bereavement brought.

Opening a blank tab in Blogger, I worked on my first post for my chosen healing technique for January.

At first, Nick and I went to therapy together, but by the end of January, he went back to work, and I went weekly on my own. It had been comforting for him to sit next to me on the couch. However, I settled in better to being the client without him there. Opening an extra cushion somehow opened more space for my thoughts. I'd been sitting across from Anna by myself for a few sessions when, after taking a sip from her steaming cup of orange jasmine tea, she asked, "How do you plan on parenting Nora?"

I raised one eyebrow in response. Had she forgotten the reason I was in her office on a freezing Friday in January? The idea of continuing to parent my stillborn baby seemed a little too silly and sentimental for me. I was craving ways to connect with Nora, but I wouldn't call it parenting, which was the act of raising Nora over time and into an adult. Parenting your dead child could be done, since at Faith's Lodge, while safely surrounded by other sad parents, I got to be Nora's mom. But doing so continually seemed excessive and even, I feared, a way to malinger in my grief.

"I don't do feelings like that," I finally replied, crossing my arms over my chest for protection from her prodding.

Anna raised an eyebrow and the corner of her mouth. "You're a therapist that doesn't do feelings?" She shot me the same neutral but knowing look she did the first time Nick and I met her. "Maybe you might want to try."

"I prefer cognitive-based, skillful interventions that aren't too emotion focused," I said smartly.

Anna let out a long, "Right," while slowly nodding her half-cocked head and then changed the subject. "What I meant by parenting Nora is . . . how do you plan on incorporating her into your life?" Anna took another sip from her mug cupped between her two hands. Her shoulders scrunched to her ears, bookending the infinity scarf encircling her neck, attempting to keep the chill of winter at bay that crept in through the windows. "Death does not have to be the end of communication with a loved one. I know you mentioned researching and writing about your experience of grief, but have you tried writing letters directly to Nora? That's more concrete and possibly 'skillful,'" she said, using an air quote. "Or is that still too touchy-feely for you as a nonfeeling therapist?"

I smiled at her sarcasm. She explained writing letters to the deceased was a way to have what the experts called continuing bonds after the death of a loved one. In 1996, grief researchers Lass, Silverman, and Nickman published a book called, *Continuing Bonds: New Understandings of Grief* that suggested a paradigm shift from the "get over grief" narrative, and instead moved toward a model that normalized the need to continue a bond with our loved one who had died.

It was okay for me to keep my relationship with Nora alive even in her death. Anna was suggesting it could even be a way for me to mother her. However, it was a shitty way to get to be a mother.

I had used the common practice of writing when working with grieving clients. They could express their emotions they might not otherwise share in talk therapy. But even though my Grief Project's healing technique this month was writing, I hadn't yet thought about penning letters about my own sorrow to Nora. I had been talking to Nora in my head nonstop since the night of her funeral, but the idea of writing her letters she would never read seemed too sad to do. Reluctantly, I took Anna's advice and bought a journal.

The brown, hardcover, pocket-sized diary had embossed emerald and sapphire flowers on the cover. Inside, the pages were lined, and a hint of vanilla lifted off them as I thumbed through and found a ruby ribbon bookmark attached to the binding. Standing between the bookshelves in Barnes and Noble, I opened the journal and knew I had to have it when I saw the backside of the cover. "This journal belongs to . . ." I imagined I'd fill it with two words not seen together often: "Nora" and "Mom."

If this diary was to be the only place where I would get to "parent" Nora, then the journal would have to be kept just for her. Running my fingers over the smooth paper inside, I promised myself to keep all my other thoughts and insecurities out of its pages. Those worries could be written on the blog. The journal would be the place where I focused only on my lost love for her.

At night, when I couldn't sleep, and my tears had drenched my pillow, I'd reach for the journal on the nightstand. Opening to a crisp, unused page with pen in hand, I wrote Nora letters longingly. It came so naturally that I'm sure grieving mothers had done so for generations . . . before the mourning mother blogs and Instagram accounts.

> *Oh Nora,*
>
> *How I wish I could have the chance to yell your name down the hall—"Nora Norine Kelly, you get down here!"—once you*

grew into a sassy teenager. But this story doesn't go that far. I'm embarrassed to admit, I used to look in my rearview mirror on my way to work while pregnant with you and imagine you there in your car seat. I would say, "Nora Kelly, you're so beautiful," in a funny, high-pitched, parent voice.

I just love the way your name sounds. Did you know that your name means "honor"? I guess I didn't know when naming you that honoring you is all I would be able to do. Darling, how I miss you. Don't worry honey, even though we don't walk this earthly plain together, I still love you and will forever. However, now I must love you from afar.

Love Always and Forever,

Mom

When I wrote Nora's name in the journal for the first time, I cried again. In that space, I got to talk to Nora and tell her about my dreams for her that would never come true. The part about writing to her that I craved the most was signing my name at the end of each letter, "Love Always and Forever, Mom." Anna was right. The journal became the one place where I believed I was warranted to wear the title.

During therapy on a frigid February morning, Anna encouraged me to read these letters. I tried holding back the tears that fell from my chin onto the cream-colored paper, smudging the pen strokes. Struggling to read the words I'd written out loud, I felt weakened by my inability to control my tears' continual flow. After reciting the closing to my letter, "Love Always and Forever, Mom," I gripped the edges of the journal, leaving fingernail dents in its leather and pleaded to Anna, "I want the pain to stop. It hurts so much." I wiped away the salt stains on my face. Reaching for a tissue on the glass coffee table between us I continued, "Will it ever not hurt this much?" I was coming to terms with having to share my own feelings in therapy, but I was still frustrated with the never-ending nature of my laments.

Anna inhaled a deep breath and held it, as if she wasn't sure she should say what she was about to say next. "No. It won't always be like this. You'll always miss her, but the pain," she looked past me and out the frost-covered window, "will be different."

My shoulders dropped, as my spine plopped back into the cushions of the couch, expelling a sigh. I was able to find an ounce of optimism in Anna's response that some relief from this suffering might someday be in sight. But I still wanted so badly to be my before-Nora-died self—the person who had her plans and emotions organized, card cataloged, and alphabetized on the appropriate shelf. The woman who didn't need a blog to be able to control her feelings. I gazed silently off to the side of the room where a strip of sunlight broke through the blinds next to the dying potted fern, flumped over with brown leaves. It looked how I felt—defeated. I realized then that the Lindsey I used to be died the moment Nora did.

chapter 16

WORKING THROUGH GRIEF

In mid-February, about six weeks after Nora died, I went back to work, deciding not to take the full twelve weeks of leave my employer offered. Staying home in an empty house was a hurtful reminder I had planned to spend my maternity leave nursing a baby.

Going back to the office had challenges of its own. My lack of retained baby weight was mentioned to me by a not-so-tactful client.

"You look great!" the bleach-blond, middle-aged woman said. She leaned closer to me in the group therapy circle where we processed clients' difficult emotions about being newly sober. In a raspy voice and smelling of cigarette smoke she said, "I can't even tell you had a baby."

"That's the problem," I mumbled under my breath so she couldn't hear my meanness through the polite smile I flashed in her direction. I was one of those envied women who didn't have to wear her maternity clothes back to the office after giving birth, unlike other loss moms, who had the added grief of wearing their pregnancy clothes postpartum with no newborn in their arms to cover the cruel reality of a leftover baby bump.

My woe was the opposite. I fit into my pre-pregnancy ward-robe. Underneath my dark-denim skinny jeans, blouse, and fitted suit jacket, my body had no marks of motherhood. No extra pounds sagging around my middle, no stitches that formed into a C-section scar, no badge of honor stretch marks on my breasts, belly, or butt, not even a fading linea nigra line. Nothing showed Nora was ever inside of me. My body betrayed her existence and my motherhood by wiping itself clean of any scars or marks left in her memory. To make matters worse, I started menstruating again the week I returned to work. My body was putting a period, literally and figuratively, on Nora's chapter in my life.

My lunch break was no break from awkwardness. While eating a bowl of soup in the breakroom a fellow therapist with two teenage daughters took a seat across from me at the table. Shifting her silver hair over her shoulder, she smiled sweetly in my direction and made small talk about our miserable Mid-west winter and office gossip. After a moment of uncomfortable silence, "One day it will happen," slipped from her lips. "You'll be a mother."

Spoon still suspended in midair, my mouth remained wide longer than intended until I remembered to act normal, sipping my spoon, full of chicken noodles and swallowing in an effort to hide my shock, as her words unknowingly crushed my soul.

I wasn't a true mother in the eyes of women like her, the non-bereft mothers. In my own therapy, I was learning there were many secondary losses piled on top of the initial one. Nick and I didn't just grieve Nora, we also grieved what we had hoped to be. First words and first steps, birthdays and baseball games, and because we didn't have other living children, our identities as parents. No "Mommy and me yoga classes," "Daddy's little girl," onesies, or easy answers to, "Do you have children?" It all evapo-rated with our daughter's death.

Things got worse as the first week of work went on. In my one-on-one therapy sessions, every hour on the hour, I had to relive a very shortened version of my story that was considered self-disclosure appropriate for the client-therapist relationship. Even though I wanted to, I couldn't hide from having this conversation with my clients. The last time they had seen me, my belly was bursting from below the breastbone. Sitting on the tweed loveseat across from my therapist chair, clients didn't know how to respond when I told them my baby died. Which made sense, since therapy was meant to be about their struggles, not mine. Each client reacted differently. Some cried, others gave me considerate condolences but most, uncomfortable, gazed out the window behind me. Unfortunately, this did not distract them from death since the view from the couch was of a cemetery in the heart of Minneapolis. Everywhere I went, Death's long shadow loomed large over me, just like new mothers and their newborns seemed to surround me at work, backing me into the corner of my office, like cats trapping a mouse.

During those first few days back at the office, a client in her early twenties, recovering from substance abuse during her pregnancy, brought her baby boy to group. *Why me?* I asked the universe in my head as a cluster of clients coincidentally had corralled outside my open office door cooing at the new mother's healthy baby in his car seat. *Why did my baby die and hers lived when I did everything painstakingly "right"?*

Not that I wanted anything bad to happen to my client's child or that I thought I was more deserving than her to birth a healthy baby. I guess I still childishly held onto a belief that since I had played by all the pregnancy rules—don't eat lunch meat or raw cookie dough; quit caffeine; abstain from alcohol; avoid soft cheese and plastics with BPA; forgo sushi; and steer clear of illegal substances—everything was supposed to work out in my favor.

"Why us? Why Nora? Why me?"

Anna didn't respond. Frost fixed to the windows that kept February's freeze on the other side of the glass, but my body was heated with anger at fate's unfairness. "Why did Nora have to die?" I was finally asking out loud the question that had been echoing in the chambers of my mind since the moment I heard the words, "no heartbeat." *Why my baby?*

It's not like I signed up for this kind of suffering, although a part of me thought maybe I did. Maybe, before I came to earth, somewhere in the ether Nora and I made a soul contract to suffer together . . . to help each other reach some level of spiritual awakening. Was I supposed to learn something (I didn't know what exactly), and she needed to complete the cycle of reincarnation? I read on a blog about a bereaved mother who went to a psychic who said stillborn babies were souls who were in their last life before they reached nirvana. They only experienced love in the womb. In some way, this made sense to me. If Nora and I made a soul contract to suffer together in this life, it meant my feelings of somehow knowing she was going to die must have been true.

"Maybe," I hesitated, letting out a deep, weighted sigh, "I could have saved her if I would have paid attention to the universe's warnings."

Anna wrinkled her forehead as she rested her head in her hand. "Like what?"

"The voice in the woods the last day she was alive saying, 'remember this,' the online forums about membrane stripping, the hesitation when cutting the tags off her baby clothes, and Nick's dream." I listed off all the "what if's" that played in my mind like a playlist stuck on repeat.

"That's called magical thinking." Anna explained. "The universe doesn't work that way. Correlation," she held out her left hand to one side and her right hand to her other, "does not equal causation," and shook her head. "Thinking about something happening doesn't mean it's going to happen or that you caused it to happen."

My stomach felt like it was in a knot, and I was trying to untangle it by fixating on my assumptions. "Then maybe it's because I wasn't grateful. Even in the days before she was born, I complained about being pregnant and uncomfortable instead of paying attention to her. Maybe if I did, she would still be alive. Maybe her dying is the universe's way of saying I don't deserve to be a mother."

Anna scooched to the tip of her overstuffed chair and leaned closer. "That's magical thinking," she said with an exaggerated sarcastic emphasis on each word.

"Well," I shook my head with sassiness and a shoulder shrug, "then I have a lot of it," understanding then why Joan Didion titled her book with a whole year of it.

Really the true answer to "Why me?" was "Why not me?" Why should I be immune to the misfortunes the universe handed out? I had lived a fortunate life up until that point. I'd been more blessed compared to others who had suffered greater tragedies, like one of my clients often said in session, "It's not like I'm a child soldier." I could relate to the reflex of wanting to compare pain, but should we?

Bereaved moms also fought in the dreaded mommy wars. We may not have been able to feud over which way to feed our baby was best, but we still managed to measure each other's pain by the yardstick of our own losses. Was a miscarriage less difficult than a stillbirth? Was a stillbirth less devastating than infant death? Which was more tragic, suddenly losing your six-week-old in his sleep or watching your six-year-old daughter die of cancer? Was one a better fate than the other and should we even equate? It seemed pointless to compare pain, which happened to be number seven of my Grief Commandments. Doing so only negated everyone's wounds.

Awkward conversations with clients aside, I enjoyed being back at work as their therapist. I looked forward to focusing on other people's pain to take the edge off mine. Maybe it was avoidance, just another way for me to sidestep grief. Maybe it was control, as it was nice being back in the therapist chair and not on the client couch. Whatever the reason, focusing on their suffering made me feel less alone in my sorrow. The universe wasn't playing favorites.

Nick thought so, too. He shared a story about a bereaved mother in the Dalai Lama's book *The Art of Happiness* that he had recently read. A woman named Kisagotami suffered the death of her only child. Desperate in grief, she went to the Buddha for medicine to bring her boy's lifeless body back to life. The Buddha said he knew of such medicine but would need a handful of mustard seeds to make it. Before the grieving mother left in search of the seed, the Buddha added the ingredient must be given from a household where no child, spouse, parent, or servant had died. Kisagotami agreed and went from house to house in search of the magical seed only to be turned away when asked if anyone had died. All answers were "yes." The mother let go of her child's barren body, realizing she was not alone in her longing.

"That's a good way to explain grief. I'm glad you find it helpful." I leaned against the sink, drying dishes that Nick washed.

"It reminds me I'm not the only one who has experienced something so devastating," he added.

I nodded and flashed him a quick smile while wiping water out of a to-go coffee cup. I secretly wondered if the Buddha had to come up with a story to justify suffering since there was so much of it.

◢◢◢

After a month back at work, my clients, co-therapist, and I sat in a circle in our clinic's conference room, its walls decorated in dated 1990s feminist artwork. We talked about weekly sober struggles, but I fought to focus. It took me twice as long to process information than it had previously. Even understanding and finding commonly used words suddenly became a struggle. I learned grief caused the "bereaved brain," but I also had pregnancy and postpartum brain, too, causing me to space out instead of staying tuned into clients' confessionals. Thankfully, my short-in-stature and in-hairstyle co-therapist, Rachel, who had been in recovery for many years herself, facilitated most of the conversations in the group. She stood at the whiteboard, stretching to reach it as she taught clients about healthy coping mechanisms to counter their addictions.

Writing, my coping mechanism, was the only place my foggy grief brain seemed to work. While clients discussed sober dates and relapses, I scribbled first drafts of blog posts on a legal pad balanced on my lap for everyone to plainly see, not caring if my coworker or clients noticed I wasn't paying attention to their problems as I frantically scribbled about my own.

If I wasn't sitting one-on-one with an individual client in my office as the sole witness to their heartaches, I lacked the empathy to care about anything outside of my own wounds. I replaced all other work time with writing. I wrote when I should have been taking notes or listening in staff meetings. I uploaded blog posts for February's healing focus—"Blogging through Grief"—when I should have been doing paperwork. I wrote at night when I couldn't sleep, and on nights when I should have been sleeping. I was as addicted to writing as my chemical health clients were to their drug of choice, and just like them, the only time I could handle my suffering was when I was immersed in my addiction.

By the end of March, having been back at the clinic for a little over two months, I was exhausted. I had hoped my therapist coworkers would have become a part of my March Grief Project healing technique of "Finding Friends in Grief" by being a support for me in my mourning. Instead, I found myself scared of being vulnerable with others at work, and I answered the everyday greeting from coworkers and clients of "How are you?" with a lie and a smile. Keeping myself together while being a support person for other sufferers of sorrow and pretending in front of my coworkers that I was functional, had eroded my armor. All I wanted to do was collapse upon the battlefield of grief, let down my shield, succumb to mourning's brutal blows, and weep.

After an afternoon team meeting on one of those draining days, I stopped by my program supervisor's office. I wanted to speak to Sarah about a concern regarding a client's recent relapse. Sarah sat at her desk with her hands on the keyboard typing when I opened the door, and she invited me in. She was dressed conservatively but in a bright, colorful, blue button-down cardigan and a red pencil skirt worn over black tights. Before the door closed behind me, she said, "I know you went through a tragic loss, but you're not present."

My muscles tightened. I felt resentful that she got to sit there with her two healthy living toddlers at home and tell me she knew what I'd been through while in the next breath saying she expected me to be fully present. My jaw clenched hard against my molars. "I'm not going to be fully present."

"I need you here," Sarah said, emphasizing the "here" with her finger pointing toward her desk. Her face was soft but, in my grief, I only saw it as stern. Nodding her head toward me, she signaled she was waiting for me to reply.

Defensive, I folded my arms across my chest. "I think I'm doing pretty well for someone in my situation."

Sarah lifted a manicured eyebrow in response, "Well, when it impacts work, I need to address it."

Angry, mostly at myself for feeling like I had failed at work as another secondary loss, I projected my frustration onto Sarah, wrongfully. I took a deep breath, and my chest trembled.

"I'm not going to be the same person I was before."

"I know. I don't expect you to be."

Really? It sounded like you're expecting me to be. My lip quivered.

She was right, though. I wasn't fully present. I had messed up a few times in staff meetings, been distracted in individual sessions, interested mostly in myself, and performing less than 100 percent as a group therapist. But I was trying to be okay with that because it felt like 50 percent or possibly more of me was missing.

Sarah continued, filling the stale space in her office left by my silence. "Are you upset Ava is pregnant?"

"Who is Ava?" I tried to relax the tension in my face.

"The new therapist. In the meeting today."

I threw my hands up, exasperated. "I've never thought about it," I retorted. "There are like three pregnant people at work, and it seems like every client has a newborn they bring to group. I'm used to it."

She squinted at me, tilting her head to the side, her curly brown bangs bouncing against her brow. "Are you sure you're ready to be back at work?"

My eyes filled with wetness I didn't want her to see. It was barely ninety days since Nora had died. I was meant to only be working for a few weeks instead of a few months by then because I should have had a newborn at home. "I don't know how to answer that," I snapped back at her.

Sarah exhaled, softening her tone. "I just need you to be more present." But it was too late. I had no desire to meet her halfway. She was now officially an evil villain in my book, even though she was just doing her job.

"I'm doing the best I can."

Her eyes looked up at me through the space between her forehead and glasses. "You're a good therapist," she tried to assuage. "But I need you *fully* present."

Determined to end the conversation, I smothered my sniffles. "I don't think I will be fully present for a while. If you notice a problem, will you let me know?"

"Yes, I will," she said, nodding her head, "and you do the same."

I walked away; fists clenched. Tears dripped down my cheeks and onto the hallway carpet.

Overcome with rage at myself, at the situation, and rightfully or wrongfully, with Sarah, I closed my office door and called my sister.

She listened to me complain through sobs and said, "What you're going through is hard. Not everyone is going to know how to respond in the way you need and that sucks. I'm sorry."

After hanging up with Kristi, I sensed I was more settled and opened my office door. Sarah had left work; her car usually parked under my window was gone. Only deep tire divots remained in the dirty snow. Relieved, I sat down at my desk to finish up notes when a soft sound of a baby's cry drifted up the stairwell from the lobby and into my office. My typing fingers froze as my heart sank. Closing my eyes, I tried rescuing the part of me inside that was drowning. After a forgotten moment, I blinked hard and regained awareness that my feet still worked. In what felt like levitating, I moved to close the door and block out the agony of hearing the infant's echo.

With my back against the hardwood and my hand still on the handle, I realized why the cry shook my core. Because I never had it. Nora had never made a sound.

Crumbling to my knees, I crawled onto the client couch where I wept uncontrollably—a grief burst—when sorrow suddenly flooded me. I wailed ugly tears into the cushions, shoving my scarf into my mouth to muffle their roar. I wasn't doing well, I finally admitted to myself. I was trying the best I could, but I was barely surviving. Grief and I wrestled daily as it fought to inhabit my body, like cancer consuming every cell. I didn't want grief and at the same time all I wanted was grief, because grief was all I had left of her.

chapter 17

NO MUD,
NO LOTUS

It snowed on and off into April. Winter, like our grief, was unwilling to leave. Outside Anna's office, green tulip stems struggled to sprout from below the snow-covered mud. The soil's earthy scent reminded me of when I was six and our family had moved into a newly built two-story home on four acres of land. That first spring, fresh rains drenched the rearranged dirt, not giving the grass a chance to take root in our front yard. One afternoon, the neighbor boys, a year or two older than I, rode their bicycles up our gravel driveway, crossing through our yard to get to their house on the other side. They landed in the slowly sinking quicksand of our grass.

Once in the mud pit, they couldn't move, stuck knee deep in the swamp. The more they struggled to free themselves, the farther the mud dragged them into its slippery soil. It seemed the ground wished to swallow them whole. I yelled for Mom in the kitchen. She ran to the garage and grabbed two two-by-fours. She placed one halfway on the gravel driveway with the other end sticking out into the muddy mire toward the boys. Walking out onto the lumber laid, Mom carefully placed the other piece of plywood on the other side of the first.

The boys moved slowly toward their wooden life raft, fighting against the riptide of the mud. They crawled on their bellies to reach the lumber and stuck their hands elbow deep into the dirt to retrieve their bikes from Mother Nature's clutches. When they finally freed themselves and their bicycles from the mud pit, they stood before us on the driveway covered in dark sludge. Only their faces were not fully afflicted, but their cheeks and foreheads were streaked with smears of dirt. The three of us watched as they struggled to maneuver their bikes, even though they were no longer in the thick of the pit. The mud had made them slow and stiff, sticking to the spokes of their wheels, jeans, T-shirts, and skin as they tried to pedal away.

I now felt the same, weighed down by mourning's muddy grasp. Emerging from the depths of the early days of sorrow, grief's menacing mud was still caked to my skin. I tasted it in my mouth, saw it underneath my nails, and felt it in the creases of my palms. When I tried wiping it away or washing it off, it remained. I couldn't get rid of it, no matter how hard I scrubbed.

In our session, I thought about telling Anna about mud as an analogy for grief until I imagined her response being, "No mud, no lotus," referring to the Buddhist proverb about suffering. But I was not yet ready to hear about possible post-traumatic growth from Anna. Instead, she brought to my attention the problem I had as a therapist seeing a therapist: I couldn't stop playing one. Anna reminded me how I tried to control the direction of the discussions, pushed back on her suggestions, and preferred to use my reasoning mind when she asked, "How does that make you feel?"

"How is the support group going?" Anna asked, slightly changing the subject.

Playing with a small pile of thread on her sofa, I said, "I stopped going."

With raised eyebrows and a "hmm," Anna nodded just once. "May I ask why?"

"It just wasn't for me." I scrunched one shoulder to my ear. "Too big of a group, maybe." It *was* too big of a group and too far away, adding another hour and a half onto the day. Those were the reasons I told myself, but really, I was embarrassed by the truth. March's Grief Project healing technique of "Finding Friends in Grief" didn't lead to new friends.

Anna tapped her thinking finger against her face with a smile that enhanced her catlike eyes. "Or maybe you had a hard time giving up control?"

I really wished I could have been my own therapist.

When I wasn't in therapy grappling with grief or hoping to read and write my way quickly through mourning, Nick and I trained for a half-marathon. The rhythm of Nick's pace bounced off the gravel road in sync with my heavy panting as we ran down the frosted wooded park path together. Every muscle of my body ached as my mind grew weaker with each step. April's Grief Project healing technique was "Sitting with Grief," and even though Nick and I weren't technically sitting still, running while grieving felt like meditating on grief. For both in running and meditating, I was left alone with my thoughts thundering through my mind. I often wished I could finish the last few minutes of meditation sessions by speeding them up like I did the last few minutes of my jogs. But on the snow-spotted gravel path, out of shape, not having run for over a year because I had been pregnant, I could not speed up my current pace, and I couldn't speed through my grief.

I only committed to completing my first half-marathon four months postpartum because I thought exercising again would help me heal my broken connection with my body and put into practice part of my fifth Grief Commandment of nurturing myself physically while mourning. But as the days until the race got shorter and our runs got longer, training felt more like punishing my body than caring for it, which is maybe why I agreed to do the run—a subconscious but socially appropriate way for me to flog my own body for its unforgivable act of not saving my baby.

"Can't you find a path without snow?" I yelled up to Nick between gulps of cool air from a few lunges behind him. He waited for me to catch up, exhaling his own cloud of fog above his head. Once by his side, I rested, bent over with my hands on my knees, trying to breathe.

"There's a paved path just around the corner," he said with his hands on his hips. His chest heaved underneath his thermal long-sleeve shirt before he continued. "Listen, Lindsey, I run for a challenge—"

I waved my mittened hand to cut him off before he could finish while the other supported my bent-over body. "Just go."

He waited, looking ahead down the path and then back at me, wondering what he should do, worried he might make the wrong choice. "Take my headphones," he said, extending his arm toward me. The white wires dangled from his gloved hand as a peace offering and a compromise.

"I don't want them," I said, irritated. "Just go."

"Are you sure?" His face contorted with concern.

"Go!" I huffed this time. He jogged off. The sound of his sneakers hitting the pavement drifted off as he distanced himself from me. I frowned, standing there while his word "challenge" reverberated between my ears. Trotting far behind him, I thought, *Haven't we had enough challenges? Why are we out here creating more obstacles for ourselves by running six miles on a rainy, muddy day in April, preparing for a half-marathon in two weeks? This was stupid, even if it was a part of my silly Grief Project.*

My feet grew heavier with every forward movement. My mourning always seemed a step ahead of me, never behind. My muscles weakened and wobbled on the trail, and so did my emotional scaffolding. Months of grappling with deep and unwanted emotions I had refused to embrace exhausted me. Panting through tears, I realized that even though I was going to therapy, writing, and reading about grief, I still tried to resist its grasp.

Understanding this didn't miraculously change me. The next week on Anna's couch, I struggled to suppress my sniffles as we discussed how unfair it was that Nora had to die before she could live. She asked her usual, "How does that make you feel?" and I avoided answering by looking out the sunlit window.

Anna paused as usual in our familiar game of tug of war. I pushed emotions away while she sat in silence, tucked confidently into the back of her chair, attempting to pull emotions out of me. "Would you just let yourself lose your shit?" she finally said. "Just lose it. This is hard. It sucks. Feel it and stop trying to control it. Stop trying to make it fit into some nice grief list with boxes you can checkmark once completed. It's not linear. It's messy and chaotic. Lose your shit so you can accept it." She paused again, like she did when she was serious. "Imagine how you might feel if you did?" Anna was paraphrasing psychologist Tara Brach from her book *Radical Acceptance,* "What would it be like if you could accept life—this moment—exactly as it is?"

Excruciating. That's what it would be. I was afraid that if I accepted grief, grief was all there would ever be. I didn't share my fear with Anna. Instead I pushed, "I don't want it. Why would I accept it?"

"In accepting it, welcoming it, you can move through it," Anna replied. Her answer reminded me of Rumi's poem *The Guest House,* about how human emotions are like visitors, sometimes unwanted. "Welcome them all! Even if they are a crowd of sorrows, violently sweeping your house of its furniture . . ."

I didn't want to invite grief in. I needed to barricade my back against my guest house door because it saved my furniture and feelings from flying across the room. But my shoulders were weakening from weeks of bracing against grief's blows. I felt slightly relieved at the idea of giving up the daily fight. But I wouldn't because I believed if Grief were allowed in, it, like Death, would never leave.

Watching the spring sunshine glint off the windowpane, I said sadly, "I birthed Death, and now all I have left to raise is Grief."

Anna nodded in agreement and shrugged. "Maybe."

Nick and I visited my family in Wisconsin two weeks later to run the Parkinson's Half-Marathon. My uncle Bobby, married to my aunt Debbie Sue, was in his fifties and had founded the race two years prior raising money to combat the degenerative disease he had been diagnosed with in his midthirties—another sad example of how suffering gets spread around.

Nick and I stood beside each other at the starting line, trying not to step in squelchy mud puddles that smelled of boggy water. We bowed our heads in silence along with all the other runners for the victims of the recent Boston Marathon bombing five days earlier, where hundreds were injured, sixteen lost limbs, and three people, including an eight-year-old boy, lost their lives. *The universe can really stop serving up pieces of its shit-filled Buddha's "life is suffering" pie*, I thought, looking at my already mud-stained tennis shoes.

After hearing the starting pistol pop, Nick and I moved forward behind the herd of other runners. We jogged the first mile together and then agreed to split off from each other to avoid arguing like we had while training. We each needed to set our own pace, as we had learned we needed to do while mourning.

All the grief books I'd been reading said that men and women grieve differently, proving true for us. While I used writing and therapy, Nick kept his emotions clutched to his heart while he ran, either away, with, or through grief. I wasn't sure which.

Only four miles into the course, I regretted my decision to run the race. My muscles were sore from the overexertion, and my mind lacked the mental fortitude to complete it. Despite my desire to desert, I settled into a kind of slow shuffle like that of the tortoise who matched the hare. My slow and steady wouldn't win this race, but I hoped it would finish at least. I slogged along like a snail for the next two miles.

My muscles and bones began to hurt around mile seven. I had difficulty breathing; my lungs aching for air were at odds with a throbbing stitch in my left side, both bidding for relief. I wanted to give up at mile nine and a half. *This is good enough,* I thought, but then I heard my inner self yelling, *Lindsey, this run is a metaphor for your life since Nora's death. You just must put one foot in front of the other and keep going. You can do this! This is nothing compared to the agony you run with every day.* For the next half mile, I forced my body to keep its turtle trot.

At mile ten, the physical and emotional discomfort had become unbearable. My toes tingled, my lungs couldn't find air, and my body was cold from the dampness of the dewy day. I decided this race, like life, sucked. I wasn't going to finish in any decent time, and I wasn't going to outrun grief, so why bother? Wishing the mud puddles on the trail would open and swallow me like the mud pit in our front yard once did for the neighbor boys, I wanted it to be over, like I wanted my grief to be over.

While walking past the eleventh mile marker, instead of hearing my own inner voice again, I heard a child's voice.

"Mom, I believe in you. You are the bravest person I know."

Tears filled my eyes. I looked up to the sky to keep from crying, thinking it might work as I was told it did as a child to keep one from sneezing. Eyes lifted to the sun poking through leftover rain clouds. Three birds sat on a branch above me. I fell to the ground on my knees where I wept, relieved for my snail's pace, since there was no one else around to see me kneeling in a puddle of mud or the puddle of grief I had become. Birds reminded me of Nora, ever since we had seen them at the lodge when we placed her stone. Seeing those three sparrows somehow confirmed the childlike voice in my head was not my own. It was Nora, saying, "I'm still with you."

After resting for a moment longer in the musty mud, I finally stood up. I could dig deep and find the strength to jog through the physical and emotional pain, or I could give in and walk the rest of the way. Or maybe it wasn't a choice between the two. Maybe it was *both* accepting the pain *and* digging deep to move through it.

It was then I realized grief was like running, the only way out of it was into it and through it. To quote Robert Frost, "The best way out is always through." This was what Anna was trying to tell me, and what my ninth Grief Commandment was about. My pain was a part of me that needed to be invited into my home to rest for a while before it could leave. It had something to say. Grief wasn't my enemy, it was just love turned inside out.

I put one foot in front of the other. My new pace was even slower, and my wet knees only added to my physical discomfort. My legs wobbled, but instead of being in constant confrontation with the pain, I embraced it, which made each step easier to make.

A tenth of a mile before I reached the finish line, I saw Nick with a completion medal around his neck. When I waved at him, he jogged to my side so we could cross the finish line together. Smiling at him, he smiled back and without a word, we both sprinted to the end.

After recovering from the race with a bottle of water and a banana, Nick and I walked to my cousin Tasha and her husband Grady's house two blocks away. Flying high from finishing a grueling thirteen miles in two hours and forty-three minutes (the time it takes a professional runner to finish a full marathon) and feeling like I received a "hello" from Nora, I dropped into sudden dread, as we knocked on the old farmhouse front door. We had to meet baby Quinn.

Quinn will forever be fixed in my mind as the baby who was born two weeks before Nora died—the child I would spend the rest of my life watching in wonder as his mom posts about the milestones he reaches on social media. Ones Nora would never get. Each new school year, I would be caught off guard by photos in my Facebook feed of Quinn standing on the front porch as he posed for pictures of the first and last day of preschool and then going off to kindergarten.

Tash and Grady welcomed us into their quaint living room, decorated in eco-friendly Pottery Barn decor. I took a seat on the couch in front of Quinn, who was in his car seat dressed in a baby GAP outfit. He was adorable with big blue eyes, dimpled cheeks, and a baby powdered scent I caught a whiff of from two feet away. I wanted nothing to do with him.

"Do you want to hold him?" Grady dressed in a windbreaker asked Nick.

Nick surprisingly said yes and reached out to receive a baby that wasn't ours. I noticed my breath shrink and go shallow with sudden dread, my heart pounding faster under my many sore muscles. Grady passed Quinn into my husband's hands, and I watched Nick bobble the baby back and forth with a burp cloth over his sweaty shoulder while my heart swelled with sadness. *This is what four months old looks like*, I thought, as I witnessed Quinn wrap his tiny five fingers around my husband's larger one. I tried envisioning Nora at that age, against Nick's chest, but couldn't. The thought was too tender to touch.

Quinn smiled up at Nick. Grady, the proud father, chuckled as he took a picture of the two with his phone. Seeing Nick, a bereft dad holding someone else's breathing baby made me wonder how the universe could be so cruel or if it was all just random.

After posing for the photo, Nick handed Quinn gently back to Tash, who smiled wide with parental pride as she bounced baby Quinn back to sleep in her arms. No one mentioned holding him to me. They seemed to have sensed I didn't want to. And they were right. I would go on to not hold another newborn until I had my own breathing baby in my arms. It was a silent promise I made to myself when I gave Nora to the nurse who took her to the morgue.

Our family of three—only two of us that you could see— said goodbye to the happy new family of three you could see and headed back to my parents' house. When we parked in the driveway, I got out of the car and walked slowly past the front yard where the neighbor boys once sank into its soil. It was currently covered in small spots of fresh green grass trying to sprout against sections of stubborn, suffocating snow.

Once inside, I soaked my sore muscles in the tub, and scrubbed the mud off my feet. I worked to scour out the dirt from under my toes, but it persisted, remaining caked onto my cuticles, causing me to cry. This time I did not resist grief's arrival and let myself sob. Letting go of my soapy washcloth, I released my bent leg from my hand, mud still under my toenails, and slowly allowed myself to sink into the warm water and into my sorrow.

chapter 18

TRYING
TO CONCEIVE

About a week after the half-marathon, I sat in my office chair during a client's canceled session and stared out my second-story window streaked in streams of rain, watching a funeral procession taking place in the cemetery across the street. White and yellow rectangular tarps covered freshly dug yet still-empty graves that spotted the cemetery this time of year. Loved ones had waited through the winter months for the snow to melt, the frozen soil to thaw, and the warmer weather of spring to arrive before they could deliver their departed's cold bodies into the ground. Black umbrellas popped open from parked cars and congregated around a headstone, keeping mourners dry from the rain above, but below their umbrellas, I imagined their faces were dripping with the wetness of their own tears.

My mind floated back to the memory of a similar damp day in April, just a year ago, when I was expectant with life, and a different type of tears wet my face after I announced to Nick I was pregnant with Nora on the day we moved into our first home. But a year later, it seemed as if life was standing still. Nothing tangible had changed. The new nursery remained unused, our new house remained silent, my new clients were still discussing their old struggles, and winter was again refusing to leave. Brushing tears off my cheeks with the scarf encircling my neck, I let out a long low sigh and sunk into my desk chair.

Still staring out the window, I noticed a baby bird trembling in a barely green tree sprouting up from the boulevard below. Pulling my chair forward with my shoeless, sock-covered feet, I inched closer to the glass and rested my chin on my arms folded into the hard window's ledge. For over an hour, after all the black umbrellas and their mourners had returned to their cars and left the cemetery in a line, I was still waiting for the sparrow with fluffy fledgling feathers to take flight. If the tiny helpless bird attempted to spread out her barely formed wings to fly, she might fall and possibly not survive. My stomach churned with anticipation, for I had something in common with that scared little sparrow. I, too, was contemplating taking a leap of faith of my own: trying again for another baby.

Nick and I had started the discussion of having a second child the day after Nora died. In the weeks and days after Nora's death, once my gynecologist gave the thumbs up for more than foreplay, I craved sex. Sex seemed to be the opposite of death to me. It was innate. A natural need for life to continue. I viewed sex as an act of defiance to death—a declaration of being alive. Back then, my mind and my heart weren't emotionally ready for another pregnancy, like the baby bird in the tree outside my office window didn't seem emotionally ready for flight.

After four months of missing Nora, Nick and I had slowly come to the agreement that our desire for another child started to outweigh our fear of losing another baby. When April approached, we weren't ready to try again, but we knew we didn't want to wait any longer to add to our family. We wouldn't try to, and we wouldn't *not try* to get pregnant.

It was only my first month of TTCing (trying to conceive), but every day for the month of April, I engaged in an alphabet soup ritual of noting my CD (cycle day), inspecting my CM (cervical mucus), and peeing on OPKs (ovulation predictor kits) to find out when my fertile window was peaking. In a day or two, postcoital, I would keep track of my DPO (days post ovulation) and settle in for the TWW (two-week wait). I counted the days on the calendar in my app for an EDD (estimated due date) and crossed my fingers for a BFP (big fat positive) while worrying if I POAS (peed on a stick) I would get a BFN (big fat negative) and be visited by AF (Aunt Flow). This alphabet soup of trying to conceive was familiar to me, as Nick and I had attempted for six months to get pregnant before I got a BFP with Nora. But this time around, it seemed more dense and harder to swallow, when doing so after the death of our baby.

The small sparrow was gone. I had missed her launch while I planned out my month's cycle. Hesitant to look down and check the sidewalk to search the concrete for clues of the sparrow's success or failure, I squeezed my eyes shut.

Cautiously, I opened one eye and peeked down two stories, when to my surprise, there was no baby sparrow in sight. Instead, a ray of sunlight shined through parted rain clouds above, creating sparkles in the pools of water on the sidewalk below. Audibly exhaling, I flopped back in my chair as a sudden lightness overcame me and with it a slow smile, thankful the scared sparrow had successfully completed her leap of faith. Maybe, it was time for me to take mine.

Arriving home from work early in the evening, I was welcomed by Georgie, who pawed at my knee-high boots. Bending down to pat his fluffy head, I nuzzled his damp nose to mine before walking into the kitchen where I found Nick. Leaning casually against the counter, he snacked on mixed nuts from the container with the cupboard door still left open. I often found his habit irritating but then something about his annoying predictability was endearing.

"Hi, my love," he greeted me between chewing and crunching fistfuls of almonds. Still in his camouflaged military fatigues, which were always flattering, he flashed a coy smile in my direction. The corners of my mouth curled upward, and my eyes twinkled at the sight of him. I hadn't seen this familiar cool and almost carefree demeanor of his in over four months, and I wanted more of him and his ease to help quiet my ache of grief.

Dropping my purse in the middle of the kitchen floor, I moved toward him and looped my arms around his neck. Pressing my body against his, my pelvis tingled as I gently brushed my lips against his clean-shaven cheek. The taste of his salty skin mixed with the subtle hints of his aromatic aftershave, leftover from that morning, lingered on my lips. Feeling frisky and needing to take advantage of my fertile window, I whispered into his ear, "Do you want to make a baby?"

Lifting one eyebrow, a smirk swelled on his face. "I do," he replied. Sneaking up the stairs in front of him, Nick patted my rear playfully, making me giggle for what seemed like the first time in a long time, finally living up to my Grief Commandment of not hiding my joy and laughter.

Once in our bedroom, I stripped down to my panties. Every other inch of my skin was naked and exposed to the cool air, giving me goosebumps. Nick waited for me on the bed on top of the fluffy, floral-printed comforter in his snug, dark-gray jockeys, and nothing else. Lifting his eyebrows twice in enjoyment at the sight of my exposed shape, he smiled.

"Come over here." He patted his lap playfully, inviting me to climb on top of him where I eagerly straddled his slender stomach.

Pressing my hips against his hardness, he slipped his hand between the soft fabric of my cotton underwear and smooth bare bum. Wanting more, I moved my mouth onto his and moaned. A pulsating tightness grew below my belly button, working its way down to my groin. I hitched to catch my breath. Pulling away from him, my eyes saw his eyes become even with the crevice between my breast and the pendant that occupied this cavern. His hardness suddenly slipped away. Everything that was moving in the right direction abruptly ended when Nick couldn't stop staring at the dangling piece of jewelry imprinted with his dead daughter's tiny footprint.

"I'm sorry," he said sheepishly, as he rubbed his hands up and down the skin of my arms. "It's not going to happen today."

I rolled off Nick's lap when he slipped out of bed and through the bedroom door.

The French refer to climaxing as *la petite mort* or "little death." But the saying doesn't only describe sexual transcendence; the term can be used for one who feels like "a part of them died inside."

And for Nick, that was what had happened to his desire. Ever since making a baby meant no more condoms and more naughty nights, Nick seemed to be less in the mood. I assumed doing the deed was too intertwined with our dead daughter. My body had turned into the vessel in which both motherhood and death lived.

Reaching for my robe hanging behind the bathroom door, I slid my arms through each silky hole and tightly secured the strap around my waist. Back down the stairs, I found Nick standing in front of the kitchen counter again. But this time he wore just jock-eys while he ate dark chocolate chips from the bag pulled out of the baking cupboard, again left open, as he poured himself a glass of red wine.

"Is everything okay?"

"Yes, Lindsey. Nothing has to be wrong," he huffed.

Feeling defensive, I crossed my arms and leaned against the

kitchen counter next to him. My cheeks burned in anger, feeling rejected.

"It's just a lot of pressure." Nick sipped his wine from a stemless glass. "You know, to do *it,* with the intent to make another baby."

"Yeah," I let out with a sigh. My body now carried too much baggage.

Nick handed me the glass of wine; its earthy aroma wafted in the air. "I still love you," he said, kissing my forehead. "The necklace just caught me off guard. And I still want to"—he winked, and the corner of his mouth went wide—"do you?"

"You do?" I replied, looking coyly up at him.

"Oh, I do!" Once more his eyebrows did a double raise in my direction.

chapter 19

A BEREAVED MOTHER'S DAY

The grief of winter lingered into May with a surprise snowstorm arriving the week before Mother's Day. It seemed apropos that the seasons were just as confused as I was. Mother's Day begged the question again of whether I qualified as a "real" mom.

The snowy Sunday before the holiday, my mother-in-law had sent me a card for what was newly known as International Bereaved Mother's Day, designating the Sunday before Mother's Day to honor grieving mothers. Barb must have seen the Facebook posts I'd shared about the new holiday. It was a sweet gesture that I appreciated, but when I opened it, I was even more confused about where I fell in the categories of motherhood. Did I get to honor both days or just the one for the moms with dead children?

The next Sunday morning, on what was known to most as Mother's Day, despite my own despair about the holiday and my uncertainty about a claim to it, Nick attempted to erase some of the emptiness that idled in the air. I woke to Jack Johnson singing "Banana Pancakes" over the speakers in the kitchen, while the warm smell of my favorite flapjacks, chocolate chip—not banana—wafted into our bedroom.

Walking into the dining area, I saw Nick pouring cream-colored batter into the frying pan, blanketing the whole circular base, making extra-large cakes. I sat down in front of my already-filled coffee cup and admired the small bouquet of fresh flowers on the table. White daisies, green chrysanthemums, and purple asters spilled over the glass vase. A few small pink roses peeked out from the pile, too, but I was unsure if it was an intentional nod to Nora or not.

I watched as Nick flipped flapjacks out of the frying pan and into the air sans spatula. We both laughed and high-fived when one flopped opposite side up on a plate. We ate our maple syrup-covered pancakes while still in our pajamas outside on the patio where a small patch of snow left in the shadowed corner of the porch slowly melted away in the warm morning sun. I was grateful for Nick, trying to make this hurtful holiday less heavy, and for that I loved him more.

That afternoon, while Nick read on the couch, I rested in the recliner avoiding Facebook and the many Mother's Day posts, and instead visited baby loss blogs. I also learned from Katherine Lane Antolini's *Memorializing Motherhood* that Mother's Day was started in 1908 by Anna Jarvis in honor of her own mother, Ann Marie Reeves Jarvis who, like me, was a bereaved mom. With about seven of Ann's possibly eleven children dying in infancy or early childhood, I couldn't comprehend her ache. If any woman needed a day devoted to her, it was Ann. But over the past century, Mother's Day celebrations started to sway away from including bereaved mothers, as there wasn't a very big selection among Hallmark card collections for us.

Feet tucked under me on the recliner, I tried processing my confused role status by writing a blog post. My few followers were expecting it, I told myself. I struggled to write words other than, *Am I a real mother?* that rested next to the blinking bullet on the computer screen. Repetitively reading the question I had typed softly under my breath, I began to sound like the baby bird in P. D.

Eastman's children's book *Are You My Mother?* and nervously asking myself, my therapist, my fellow bereaved mama friends, and my dog. I'm pretty sure if I would have passed a cow or a crane, I probably would have asked them, too.

It didn't help that early in the week, a new and well-meaning, middle-aged client, recently in recovery from years of struggling with alcohol addiction, asked at the end of our first session, "When are you and your husband going to have children?"

This came up after she had shared tidbits of her own children with me. The client really wanted to know if I could relate to her version of motherhood and its struggles. I tensed up like a frightened rabbit in my therapist chair. My eyes, like a scared bunny's dark beady ones, darted in all directions for a possible place to flee but there was none. Instead, I quickly pondered my response. I had three options:

1) I could be honest and tell her I had a baby, but she died. My client then, feeling uneasy, would never come back for a second session.

2) I could be half honest and tell her I have a daughter. My client then would ask further questions like my child's age, and I would become baffled about how to reply, eventually telling her my baby died anyway. Things would become awkward.

3) I could lie, telling her I'm not sure when we'll start. Saving my client and myself from any further uncomfortable conversations but doing so would leave me feeling spineless.

I wanted so badly to choose option one, but instead I heard myself reply, "Maybe someday." The blood drained from my face as I suddenly felt I didn't deserve to be Nora's mother since I didn't have the courage to claim her in the conversation. It's not that I was ashamed of Nora for being dead. It was just hard to be honest with people when they said the most hurtful things back to the bereaved.

A BEREAVED MOTHER'S DAY

♪♪♪

A few weeks earlier, I had been wandering the muddy grounds of the graves in the cemetery, secretly visiting the tombstone of another named Nora on my lunch break. My Nora was back at home in her ugly urn, but there was something nurturing about being with Nora, even if it was one from a hundred years ago. This Nora's headstone had many years between the two dates etched in the stone that still shone brightly in the spring sunlight.

While cleaning decayed wet leaves from around the grave, an elderly woman in her late eighties held the arm of a younger woman, who resembled her.

They walked by me with a bouquet of flowers in her free hand and asked, "Are you visiting someone, too?"

Feeling foolish, I nodded silently when the elder of the two continued, "I'm so sorry. Who did you lose?"

Blushing, I took a breath and decided to be honest this time. "Umm . . . my daughter. She was stillborn."

The younger of the pair gave me a look of sympathy. Her mother with silver hair said, "That makes it easier, right?"

My body warmed in anger, while standing in the shade of the old oak tree on the cool spring day. I knew to this grieving widow, who had recently lost her husband to what I imagined was many decades, that a loss like mine, where you only knew your beloved briefly, might seem to bring less suffering. I stood there in silence, frustrated that people didn't understand it's not the length of love but the depth of love that matters. Part of the pain of losing a baby was you had hardly any puzzle pieces left behind to put together a portrait of your child. Where most bereaved have memories, bereaved parents only have questions. What would her laugh have sounded like? Would she have loved princesses or pirates, or maybe both? Nora had such little time to mold into my memory.

Blinking tightly and struggling to see through the bubbling tears, I heard the daughter of the widow speak, unmistakably mortified by her mother. "I think it hurts no matter how long someone lives, Mom."

Not knowing how to respond, I kept my gaze on the ground, focusing on sidestepping mud puddles as I walked away.

Interactions like these made me question my motherhood and added to the confusion of who I was or wasn't on Mother's Day. Feeling forlorn, I peeked into Nora's nursery before bed where I found four white pages in the middle of the floor. I had left the papers there from a meditation called, "nondominant handwriting," that I did a few weekends before for April's Grief Project focus of "Sitting with Grief," after reading about it in *On Grief and Grieving* by Elisabeth Kübler-Ross and David Kessler. They suggested you ask a question to your deceased loved one in a meditative state with paper and pen in front of you and see what either your subconscious or dead loved one had to say.

I had sat on the ground in Nora's nursery in my pajamas, burrowed beneath my Linus blanket. I tried the exercise with the lights off, not wanting to wake Nick with the glow from Nora's room. Closing my eyes with pen in hand I waited, for what I wasn't sure.

Then I talked to Nora in my mind. I told her I missed her, I loved her, and I was in a lot of pain. I said I was ready to receive her answers, ready for anything to happen. I started crying. Sobbing. Streaks of sadness rolled down my face while a feeling of light filled my body, like the way it had that morning when I first awoke, the day after she died.

A drop of dampness fell from the base of my chin down to graze the soft skin of my chest. *This is where she was supposed to be, but she wasn't there.* I sobbed deep and wounded whimpers and pulled my left hand to my heart and my right, still holding a pen, over where she used to live—my empty womb. Inhaling and exhaling deliberately, I immersed myself in the wet, yet warm, ache.

Sitting there in sorrow, I heard a childlike voice call out.

"Mom." And then again, "Mom." Over and over. It was Nora once more talking to me in such a comforting way. How I hoped my future children would utter the word incessantly someday. A sad smile shifted across my fractured face.

My mind then took me to a seashore, where Nora and I danced on its bank. I heard the waves hitting the sand and felt my feet sink into its soft grains. Nora was a little girl, probably aged four. She wore a yellow maxi dress, and I was in a blue one, frolicking together on the beach barefoot. Her chocolate-colored hair was pulled back in pigtails as she and I giggled. She pointed to the waves, the sand, the sky, inquisitively asking me questions. I saw myself grinning gratefully, amused by my daughter's youthful curiosity. But in reality, I knew I sat eyes closed with tear stains underneath, next to an empty crib, imagining all this in my head as if watching a homemade movie of Nora and me.

Hearing a howl coming from somewhere on the beach, I searched for its source. Slowly, I began to understand the groan was my own. The roar left my lungs as I longed for this vision to be true.

"Why? Why can't I have you?" I asked the nursery walls. Nora, no longer on the beach but her voice in my mind, responded as I imagined a wise old soul would. "No one can have anyone, Mommy."

"You may house their bodies but not their souls," Kahlil Gibran wrote about children.

I heard myself whine mournfully as I knew this to be true.

I had a sudden nervous need to find her, to open her urn behind me on the dresser so I could see her, feel her, and hold her again. I even envisioned eating her ashes, for us to become one once more.

"You will not find me there," I heard her say. "I am here," and she showed me an image of the breeze in the trees and the stars in the sky. I cringed and cried as I knew she was right.

Placing pen to paper, I continued wailing, and my hand moved to write the message Nora needed me to read. A part of me knew it was my own subconscious comforting me. I wasn't crazy, just grieving. But I kept writing anyway, not looking at what appeared on the page. My hand moved intuitively. A darkness floated about the room. The writing stopped. The pen fell onto the paper.

"I love you. Mommy."

Feeling her drifting away, I became frightened. I shouted to an empty and dark nursery, "Don't go! Please stay!" But she was already gone.

After the vision was over, I crawled back into bed with Nick. I didn't read what I had written but left the pen and paper on the floor before going to sleep. The visit from Nora was enough.

As the week passed, I walked by her nursery and caught glimpses of the paper with scribbles laying in the middle of the room but made no effort to revisit it.

Now, on the evening of Mother's Day, I held those four white pages in my hands. They were full of scratched scribbles, most of it illegible, like a four-year-old's handwriting. Taking a seat again in the middle of the nursery floor, I attempted to read the scrawls.

Dear Mom,

I miss you, too. I love you, but I had to go. I was never meant to stay. You don't need to save me, as I didn't need to be saved. Please let me go, Mom. Let the pain go. You are a good mom. I chose you. You held me my whole life. I never felt any pain. I am only loved. I am love. I am happy, Mom. This is because I know you.

My face leaned in closer to the pages as my body became cold with chills as if frosted ants marched down my spine. I couldn't believe what I had read. I had no doubt some of those thoughts were mine, but I sensed some of them weren't, too. It *felt* like I was receiving a letter from Nora. But I also knew it could have been my subconscious, writing down what I hoped I could hear her say. Either way, it made the emptiness of the day feel slightly fuller, as if Nora and I were once again connected, even if the connection was just one-sided.

chapter 20

NO ONE WORD

Life began blooming all around us as winter eventually gave way to spring. In mid-May, my mother planted a garden in her front yard dedicated to Nora. Mom texted me ideas about the whimsical flower bed with a *Wizard of Oz* theme. There would be a yellow brick road, a scarecrow, a tin man, and Toto, too, all helping Nora, like Dorothy, find her way home. We planned on spreading part of her ashes there when it was completed at the end of summer. How I wish Mom could nurture Nora like she did her garden.

Dad didn't garden, but he sent me photos of the withered pink rose tattoo he got inked on his arm in honor of Nora. It grew out of the larger red rose on his bicep that represented me, which grew out of an even larger red rose that represented my mother. *What if she hadn't died? Would Nora's rose still be pink?* I wondered. I hadn't told my parents I picked pink roses because I hated them. I probably never would since one was permanently placed on my dad's pigmented skin.

We all mourn differently, and grandparents grieve, too. The saying, "Grandparents grieve twice," refers to the grandchild they lost and again for the pain the loss puts their own child through.

I uploaded my parents' pictures on both my blog and Instagram as the Grief Project healing technique for May was "Other

People's Grief," shifting the spotlight of sorrow from solely my mourning and onto other members in my family. It reminded me to follow my fourth Grief Commandment of not grieving alone and needing others to heal. I posted a picture on Instagram of Dad's pink rose tattoo overlaid with Mom's heart-shaped Nora necklace, adding to the many other photos posted since March.

The Instagram comment section was where I connected with the editor of *Still Standing Magazine,* an online blog for bereaved parents, and I was asked to join their team as a contributor.

Sitting cross-legged on the couch in front of my laptop, a warm, blossom-scented spring wind blew in through the window as I typed in "Child Loss" for the title of my first article I wrote for the magazine. This word combination bothered me because like most bereaved parents I didn't *lose* my child. She's not missing. I couldn't go collect her from the lost-and-found booth at the Minnesota State Fair. I knew where she was. Her ashes were in an ugly urn in her empty nursery. She was dead. Not lost, like Peter Pan's lost boys. I tapped the delete key to remove the phrase.

Bereaved parents deserve more accurate words to describe their child's death. Dead baby. Dead child. It's agonizing when using those two words together in the same sentence, but they are the truth. Maybe if we had a word for bereaved parents like we did widows, widowers, and orphans, this wouldn't be an issue. Duke English Professor Karla Holloway, a bereft mother herself, suggested in her article "A Name for a Parent Who's Child has Died" that *vilomah*, the Sanskrit word for "against natural order," should be adopted as the term for bereaved parents. But maybe a defining word has not caught on because one cannot succinctly capture the ache.

Deciding I wasn't going to be that person who used *child loss* instead of *dead child* as if we are all in Hogwarts silently uttering under our breath, "He-who-shall-not-be-named," I typed the uncomfortable phrase "dead child" into the title of my blog post and pressed submit.

No matter how soft we frame it, for those of us who must live with death daily, our harsh reality is still heavy. Our child is still dead.

chapter 21

IF ONLY
AND WHAT IF

Nick's birthday and our two-year anniversary arrived at the end of May as spring snuck into summer. We sat at the dinner table enjoying our dessert of strawberries, chocolate, and red wine as a breeze blew in the smell of fresh-cut grass through the open windows.

Nick reached for the last berry when I asked out of nowhere, "Are you mad at me for not going to the hospital that night, when I noticed Nora wasn't moving as much?" His birthday and our anniversary haunted me with the "if onlys" and "what ifs" of my grief.

Nick retracted his reach for the strawberry and found my gaze. In a somber tone, he replied with a gentle but firm, "No."

I looked away from him and down at our empty dessert dish. "But what if I would have listened to my worry like I normally do? What if I would have woken you up and insisted that we go to the hospital instead of going downstairs to get a snack, which made her move?" I bit my bottom lip as I faltered. "If only I hadn't let it falsely calm my fears."

"What time was that?"

"It was nine at night." I could never forget. It was the last time I felt her move, but the truth was, she could have already been dead.

Cadaveric spasm, also known as postmortem spasm, occurs when muscles stiffen as rigor mortis sets in.

Nick sat back in his chair; his hands folded in his lap as he took a moment to contemplate. "I don't think it would have made a difference. Even if we would have gone in then, it was probably too late. Remember what the doctor said?"

Nick was referring to the phone conversation about the autopsy report we had back in February on Valentine's Day with my gynecologist. We had both huddled over the phone on speaker at the same table where we currently sat. We had listened to the doctor review the large twelve-page document we had received in the mail. We learned the color and size of each of Nora's tiny organs; the weight and length of her body to the exact ounce and inch; the dimensions of her umbilical cord; the non-remarkableness of her placenta; the name of the bacteria, *Escherichia coli*, that killed her; and the method of its attack, ascending upward in the vaginal canal and through the two chorioamniotic membranes, the amnion and the chorion, which made up the amniotic sac that surrounded and failed to protect her. There were things the autopsy report didn't tell us, too, like the color of her eyes, the shape of her palm in mine, if she would have been right-handed or left, or if the brown birthmark the size of a dime on the bottom left of her belly was there or not. I thought I saw it for a split second before the nurses took her to be clothed. If only I would have let my eyes linger longer over her final frame, maybe then I could have remembered.

"Even if she was born alive, she probably wouldn't have survived," I replied. The seriousness of her infection in the autopsy results indicated severe pneumonia was found in her lungs. "That is the one thing that helps me deal with the guilt. But Nick, what if I wouldn't have done the membrane sweep?"

Nick drew in a frustrated breath and released it. "The doctors said that had nothing to do with why she died."

"I know, but as her mother, I feel like I should have known." I shook my head and let out a long sigh. "I second-guessed my gut. If only I would have gone in."

"You can't do that," he said shortly, tossing his napkin onto his plate. The chair legs dragged on the floor as he quickly stood from the table to put his dish in the sink. I sat still in my seat. From the moment we found out Nora had died, I kept apologizing over and over, until Nick took my hand and said sternly, with Nora still under my skin, "It's not your fault."

Not wanting to fight with him on his birthday, I slowly stood and walked toward the speaker the phone was plugged into and pressed play.

Nick turned as he heard the familiar lyrics from two years before on that day. When we held each other close and danced to the same song, "Someone Like You" by Van Morrison, the evening we exchanged our vows.

Moving toward him, I silently took his hand in mine as a soft smile budded across his face, relieved I'd let go of the conversation for the moment. Embracing, we slowly swayed back and forth holding each other as we danced around our hardwood kitchen floor. I whispered in his ear, "I'm sorry she's not here on your birthday."

"I know. Me, too."

Then we waltzed and wept, hoping, like we did on our wedding day, that our best years were yet to be.

chapter 22

WOMAN'S SEARCH
FOR MEANING

"Have you found meaning in your loss yet?" Anna asked, in a therapy session at the end of spring.

Scrunching my eyebrows and mouth together, a look of "really" radiated from my face. Anna replied with a forward head nod and a look of, "yes, really," on hers. I pondered her question while noticing the unused fireplace behind her chair—hollow, empty, and longing for a lively fire to burn within—was just like me.

Over the last few months, I had come to terms with accepting that my grief was my love for Nora trying to find a place to go, but I still didn't see any meaning to be made from her dying.

"I don't know," I said, shrugging. "If I don't believe in a God who is supposed to have a grand plan for me, then can there still be meaning in Nora's death? It's all random, right?"

Anna twirled a pen between her fingers like a magic wand I wished she could wave to help me find my answer. "Even without faith, some can still find meaning in a devastating loss like yours. It can help with the grieving process."

Trying to think of what meaning might be made from Nora's death, I crossed my arms and let my back fall into the sunken couch cushions, my thoughts drifting to a dream I had a few months after Nora died.

In the dream I was in a hospital bed, giving birth to a different baby, with Nick by my side. I looked down at my once-again swollen stomach, where a wiggly newborn could be seen through my opaque belly, like that of the San Jose Cochran frog, better known as the glass frog, whose organs showed through its translucent skin. (It's a dream, remember. Dreams are weird.) I could make out the silhouette of the baby's profile, a button nose on a round face, reminding me of Nora. But like one instinctively does in a dream, I knew this baby was not her. Through my glass skin, I could tell this baby was a boy.

When it came time to deliver, I lost consciousness, and everything went dark. I woke up, still in the dream, and I held a baby in my arms. He was a small baby, but a breathing one. "He's *alive!*" I heard myself shouting. And then I woke up.

After describing the dream to Anna, I paused before I concluded, "The only meaning that could possibly come from Nora's death would be if we were to have another child because maybe that child would not have been born if Nora hadn't died." Swallowing hard, I met Anna's eyes and choked back salty tears. I shrugged my shoulders one more time. "But even that seems unfair."

As May turned to June, summer followed its arrival, and Nick and I took a trip to France, hoping to escape grief, with June's Grief Project being "Taking a Break from Grief."

When we arrived at our hotel in Paris across the street from the Jardin de Tuileries, we unpacked our suitcases and found grief had tagged along. Mourning had settled itself into Nick's suitcase more than mine. His mood was flat as we ate chocolate crepes while walking along La Seine, strolling by Parisian pedestrians and La Louvre. Nick, unlike other tourists, was uninterested in entering. Instead, we passed by the glass pyramid entryway where tourists took photos with silent mimes and street performers who populated the area for entertainment.

The sunny, summery day later turned to drizzle, which matched Nick's demeanor. He never smiled as we climbed the medieval stone steps of the Notre Dame Cathedral. For Nick, who loved to travel, I thought this trip would create a shift in his mourning. But on the streets of Paris, we learned we couldn't flee from grief.

It follows you, like night follows day.

It had followed us across an ocean.

A few days later, we stayed in a quaint little cottage on the Normandy coast in northern France. Desperately searching for something to do, Nick paced the tiled floors of the stuffy seaside home as rain pounded against the roof. Without the internet or a book to read, Nick was left alone with thoughts and feelings he didn't want to have. It was as if he packed an itchy wool grief sweater that he wore for the entire trip. If he wiggled his shoulders beneath its starch fabric, he was unable to ignore the itch sadness needed him to scratch.

For three months after Nora's death, Nick had felt like he was on an upswing from grief. Then he stalled, with no forward or upward progress. I hadn't checked in with him recently about his sorrow because the answer was always the same.

"I feel like I hit a plateau in my mourning." His mood on our vacation confirmed he was still seated on that high hill.

For the past six months, I didn't know how to relate to Nick's feelings of stagnation, for my tenth Grief Commandment seemed to be accurate for me. "I move forward through my grief each day. It's always there, but each day it gets better." I hadn't felt stuck like him until recently, as I was beginning to understand Nick's frustration with his unmet expectations of bereavement.

When the rain had settled into a mist, Nick and I went down to the beach to alleviate his agitation. Nick stayed silent and forlorn as we walked along the sand, so I thought about my own mourning and how I assumed it would continue to wane at the same pace it had been without a resurgence of sorrow.

Early grief reminded me of the salty scented sea I had visited as a kid in Cape Cod off the coast of Provincetown. For hours, low tide continually receded to reveal the vast wet and soft sandy shore underneath. I forgot, like I did then, that high tide was known to clap back without warning, surprising unexpecting visitors like my seven-year-old self.

Trying to ignore Nick's sulking, I split off from him as we then walked the Normandy shore apart, attempting to enjoy the clouded and cold beach. I found a small stick of driftwood and wrote Nora's name in big letters, leaving deep crevices in the soggy sand, her etched name impermanent, like she was. I sensed grief's wave return, crashing on my thirty-year-old self's shore strongly again, like the sea did against the desolate coast I stood on.

On the last day of our trip, in the afternoon, we stood at the top of the Eiffel Tower under a sweltering sun that covered the city of Paris in a haze below. Nick, dressed in a short-sleeved, linen, collared shirt, finally admitted he hated the trip.

"You know it's hard being here. We wouldn't have taken this trip if Nora didn't die."

"I get that," I replied, securing my sundress against the breeze, not having much else to say. Both of us silently stood shoulder to shoulder looking out over the city that seemed to have no end as I thought of Anna's question about meaning. Maybe coming to France was the only meaning to be made from Nora's death. But the trip seemed like a weird consolation prize.

Looking back at the photos from the vacation, I saw our sorrowful eyes shining through forced smiles in our selfies. Our sadness slyly seeped past the Instagram filters. The creases on our foreheads and around our lips looked deep for such young faces. Nick's hair bore flecks of white that I swore hadn't been there in the photo taken of us that previous Christmas standing in front of our fireplace, his hand on my large belly with Nora inside. Grief had aged us.

The day after we returned home, Nick and I were out for a stroll with Georgie when I asked him Anna's question. "Have you found any meaning in Nora's death?"

Nick stared ahead down the suburban, cemented sidewalk.

"Anna asked me this before we left for France. I can't think of any, can you?"

"I don't know if this counts," Nick said, holding onto the handle of the retractable leash, as Georgie zig zagged in front of us between the freshly cut manicured lawns and the street curb. "But do you remember that book I read right after Nora died, *Man's Search for Meaning*, by Viktor Frankl?"

I nodded while watching our pup sniff in the smells of summer.

"Frankl was a Jewish psychiatrist and prisoner in the Nazi concentration camps during World War II," Nick said. "He survived and made the study of suffering his life's work. As a psychiatrist, he worked with a widower who deeply mourned his wife. Frankl asked this man, what would have happened if his wife hadn't died first and was left to grieve him instead?" Nick called for George who was sniffing tall grass around the fire hydrant.

"What did he say?"

Nick gently tugged on George's leash as we rounded the corner. "The widower answered that his wife would have suffered greatly, more than him, he assumed. With which Frankl replied,

'Suffering has been spared her because you have accepted her suffering for her.'" Nick looked at me as we waited for George to finish his marking on a stop sign. "Think about it. What if you would have died, and Nora had lived? How awful would that be to grow up without your mother? I would much rather Nora not have to suffer the grief of missing you or us, even if it means we must suffer missing her." He ended by shrugging his shoulders. "That's what this suffering means to me, I guess."

I was surprised by Nick's answer and that he even had an answer. After months of feeling like he had plateaued, even still feeling that way three days ago while we were in France, I did not expect him to have made any meaning from Nora's death. I also knew his meaning didn't magically turn it into mine, as I had hoped.

Nick kneeled on the stoop outside our front door to pet George before he took off his collar, and they both stepped inside. Anna was right about the need for meaning. Nick's was a fine example of the German classical philosopher Nietzsche's saying, who Frankl quoted, "He who has a 'why' to live can bear almost any how."

That weekend I met a fellow bereaved mama friend, Andrea, at a coffee shop. We had first connected in the online world of baby bereavement messaging boards. She was in her midthirties and sported a spunky hairstyle with thick blond bangs whisked over her forehead. She sat across from me at a small table next to a large window in the café. She drank bitter-scented coffee, while I sipped sweet-tasting chamomile tea, and we talked about our dead children. Her daughter had died of a freak choking accident while eating a carrot at two years old, four years before, and mine who at age zero had died before she was born because of a microbe.

Having read my blog, Andrea asked, "How could you share so candidly about your mourning?"

I was surprised by her question because she was a fellow writer who encouraged others like us with her words on mothering a missing child. "When I started the Grief Project, I promised myself I would not hide my grief, as I did not hide my love. It was my first Grief Commandment: 'The pain is great because the love is great.' I had come to see my grief as a battle scar I wore proudly for loving so deeply and why I wrote so openly."

Andrea gave me a silent but knowing bereaved mother nod as she sipped her cappuccino from a white ceramic mug.

Those words I spoke to Andrea over coffee were part of a post that I'd written for *Still Standing Magazine* earlier that month. Interested in revisiting what I had originally written after my coffee outing, I pulled up WordPress on my laptop and clicked on the article that was posted while we were away in Europe. It had been shared over three thousand times since we had left for France. Thousands of other mourning mothers and fathers felt the same way I did.

At my next therapy session, I was flying high with validation from other bereaved parents sharing my prose on social media and told Anna all I wanted to do was write. Offering comfort through my words to others was surprisingly comforting to me. "I wish I could spend all day blogging."

"Why?" she asked, wanting me to go deeper. Either Anna challenging me emotionally or the afternoon sun from outside the window flooding my face caused sweat to rise on my forehead.

Wiping my brow with a tissue, I exhaled deeply. "It's the only way I get to be with her. Writing gives me purpose. Like I thought I would have with her." I crumbled my tissue for a moment before continuing. "I guess that's where I find meaning. It's how I get to parent her." A silent tear rolled down the side of my nose and onto my quivering lip.

Anna sat with me in silence, radiating empathy. She created a container as it's sometimes called in therapy for me to, "feel felt." Daniel Siegel, a renowned clinical professor of psychiatry and author of *Mindsight*, coined the term to explain how empathy paired with acceptance and presence creates a holding space for deep understanding, something society often struggles to provide others, especially the grieving.

"To continue to write about her, for her, because of her, I'm able to have one more minute, one more hour, one more day with her." I sat silently under streaks of sunlight spilling in through the blinds.

The instinct of wanting to parent your child is still present even in their death. It doesn't go away when they do. The desire grows stronger. The want becomes an all-consuming need unable to be filled.

On Father's Day, I turned to writing once again to acknowledge our place as Nora's parents. I left the letter I had written to Nick on the coffee table next to him before I went into our bedroom where I stood in front of the mirror above my dresser. I decided to take off Nora's footprint necklace, which I'd worn for the past six months.

While hearing Nick's sweet sniffles sweep through the bedroom door as he read his Father's Day card on the couch, I brought the two ends of the chains together, clasping and closing the silver circle. My grief had not yet come full circle, but I was aware of a shift inside of me. The sadness was still deep, the yearning still strong, but a part of me had settled into acceptance that Nora as my living child, would never be. Placing the chain around the dresser dowel attached to the mirror, something in me said it was time to put the pendant aside. Maybe in hopes of making room for something new? I wasn't sure, but I knew I no longer needed the reminder of Nora next to my heart as a symbol of my motherhood.

She already lived there.

chapter 23

THE TWO-WEEK
WAIT

The quick pulse of my heartbeat roared in my ears on a sticky summer afternoon in early July. It was the loudest sound in the bathroom. I closed my eyes to center myself. Standing up from the toilet, I pulled up my pants and placed the pregnancy test on the edge of the sink. I checked to make sure the first "blue line" appeared, which registered I had peed on the stick properly and my result would be accurate. I had done this ritual three times in the last four months, but I still reached for the directions. "Wait three minutes until reading results."

I set the timer on my phone and watched as the seconds slowly counted backward. A lot can happen in three minutes—you can pop popcorn, have a glass of wine, make a baby, find out you're having a baby, and be told your baby had died.

I checked the timer. One minute passed.

A wave of nausea flooded me. I folded my knees onto the ground in front of the toilet and pressed my cheek to the cool tile floor for relief. I tasted the subtle hint of vomit in the back of my mouth. Was the need to gag a sign of early morning sickness or was it just nerves? I feared either answer the test might give. If I were pregnant, I would be relieved for a moment and then hold my breath for the next nine months, hoping this baby didn't die, too. If I weren't pregnant, Nick and I would be another month farther away from having another baby, needing to repeat the ritual all over again next month.

Two minutes. The numbers on the phone glowed.

I reached an arm up to the counter and checked the test. No blue line yet. From experience, I knew this wasn't a good sign. Placing the test back on the sink's ledge I returned to my kneeled position. My need to throw up suddenly dissipated and settled into a low-grade stomachache.

The timer chimed. Three minutes had passed.

Lifting the little stick to my eyes, I already knew its answer.

A BFN—Big Fat Negative—as they said in all the online baby boards. No second blue line. No positive plus sign signaling we would be adding to our family. I tossed the test into the trash. This time, unlike the previous three months before, I didn't go back ten minutes later to reach into the small bin under the sink to make sure the second line hadn't magically appeared.

"How are you feeling about trying for another baby?" Anna asked a week later in therapy. The scent of freshly-trimmed grass wafted through her opened office window along with the low hum of a lawnmower.

Trying again had become exhausting. Sex was no longer fun and was now a chore on the to-do list: run the dishwasher, write a blog post for July's Grief Project healing technique of "Remembering with Rituals," complete client case notes, walk the dog, and copulate because my basal body temperature told me it was the optimal time to do the naked tango with my husband.

I recounted to Anna our attempts at baby-making over the last four months. "I'm still mad at my body for not saving Nora." To me, my body was like Humpty Dumpty after his great fall. All the therapy and all the blogging couldn't put me back together again. "I'm not sure how I'm supposed to trust my body again with a baby when she's like a cheating boyfriend who promises, 'It won't happen again.'"

"Maybe you could revisit the letters you wrote back in February?" She was referring to the letters she asked me to write from Ms. Soul (me) to Ms. Body (my body) and then Ms. Body back to Ms. Soul. It was a therapeutic exercise that fit in well with my Grief Project's healing technique, "Blogging Through Grief," but once we tried to conceive again, there seemed to be more unresolved animosity between the two parts of me.

While walking to my car after my therapy appointment, the heat of summer caught between my thighs in the form of sweat chafing against the skin under my skirt. I had lost all the baby weight left over from being pregnant, but I still criticized myself for how my fat now distributed differently across my frame. Reaching the driver's side door before opening it, I caught a glimpse of my reflection in its tinted window. Moving my head from left to right, I examined the big nose that graced my face since I was prepubescent but it, too, seemed like it looked a little larger than before pregnancy. I still couldn't comprehend that my body was beautiful, or that I belonged in it. Even during Nora's perfect pregnancy before she died, I never really believed my body was on my side. Maybe it had something to do with my own birth story my mother told me, where my baby body almost killed hers.

The combined years of awkwardness and anguish had added up to a troubled relationship between Ms. Body and Ms. Soul, and losing Nora only solidified what I already knew to be true. My body was one of the ugly and unlucky ones.

Shutting the door to the car, I pulled up my blog on my phone to reread the original letters.

Ms. Soul was angry. Irate. Spewing words of hate and betrayal in her letter to Ms. Body. "You failed me! I trusted you with my child, and you killed her!"

Ms. Body replied in her letter, "I'm sorry. I tried everything I could to bring her into the world. I promise I did. I never meant for any of this to happen. But, Lindsey, I didn't know she was dying. And for that, I am so sorry."

Dropping my phone, I began bawling. My head was hunched over the steering wheel when I heard Ms. Body whisper, "Lindsey, I miss you. I didn't mean for Nora to die."

I nodded through tears as I heard Ms. Soul say, "I know."

"Can we grieve together? I need us to grieve together," Ms. Body begged.

I nodded again, and Ms. Soul replied, "Yes! It's not your fault. I'm ready to move forward. Together."

"Me, too," Ms. Body softly said. "Thank you for forgiving me."

In our next therapy session, a week later, I told Anna about my body and soul's conversation in the car.

"My body wanted to be a mother just as badly as my soul did. She did everything she could to save Nora." Sucking in air through parted lips, I suppressed tears. "But she had Nora stolen from her, too." Holding my face in my hands, I let out my cries not just for my soul but for my body that worked so hard to create and keep life. Ms. Body had wept with me from her breasts in those first days of mourning. She had lost Nora, too. There weren't two of us. There was only *us*, as one. My body had been grieving with me all along.

Anna explained how grief, like pregnancy, was embodied. It's not just an emotional loss, it's a physical one. It ached in your joints and moved like a lightning strike through your muscles. Our bodies grieved with every cell in our system. My body knew Nora. My body longed for Nora too.

A sudden wave of relief washed over me. My weight pushed

heavily into the cushions of the couch where I sank into its crevasses. Ms. Body and Ms. Soul merged back into one. Solid and grounded in our solidified form, a subtle sadness surfaced from within our shared being. We had gone on too long mourning without each other. But with our renewed bonding, I started to believe that together we could carry the weight of grief and possibly even a future pregnancy.

pregnant again

"Please don't take my sunshine away . . ."

—*Jimmie Davies, "You Are My Sunshine"*

chapter 24

BIG FAT POSITIVE

"I'm pregnant," I blurted out without warning to Nick who was mid sit-up on the living room floor.

My husband froze with his elbows touching his knees that hung in the humid August air. He stood and wiped away the small beads of sweat that had accumulated on his forehead during his daily training for the upcoming Twin Cities marathon.

"The test says I'm probably pregnant," as if there could be an in-between.

"Where is the test?" Nick wanted proof of my presumed pregnancy proclamation.

"It's in the trash." It had felt natural to put the fifth one where I had placed the past four, even if the result was possibly different. "You want to see it?"

He walked to the bathroom. While waiting for him to return, I remembered when I'd said the same sentence to Dr. Hayes during my first prenatal appointment with Nora.

She had chuckled then and smiled wide, showing her bright white teeth. "You either are or are not pregnant." I'm guessing Dr. Hayes had never lost a baby. Because as a mourning mother, I spent most of my time in the place in between.

Nick returned to the living room and held the pregnancy test parallel to our wishful, hoping-to-be-parents' eyes as George paced anxiously at our feet.

"That's not a line," Nick concluded. "It's too faint."

"Well according to the directions, it says, *any* line is a positive result.'"

Grimacing, he shook his head. "It's too early. You haven't even missed your period yet."

"I know," I said softly, realizing he was right. Walking back to the bathroom, I threw the test back in the trash bin under the sink. The excitement of being pregnant again had left before it had a chance to arrive. The joyful innocence of believing a positive pregnancy test would bring home a baby was gone. Hope for this new pregnancy was being held hostage by the disappointment of the previous one.

Inspecting the bottom half of my torso in the medicine cabinet mirror, I turned sideways, pulled up my gray tank top, and placed a hand on my solid stomach. No one could tell it had once held a newborn Nora or another baby within its walls. I admitted to myself I didn't want to be pregnant with a different baby. I wanted another chance to be pregnant with Nora.

And within the same second, I felt at fault for the thought, the wish of wanting Nora and not this maybe-baby. Was the longing for her to again grow there unfair to whatever life who dared to take root inside my womb? I pushed the thought away as I wasn't yet ready to find alignment with this maybe-baby over my deeply rooted allegiance to Nora. Doing so, I believed, would be a betrayal of my loyalty to loving her.

Taking a few steps out of the bathroom, I moved toward the bed and flopped face first onto the side where I no longer slept— the place I was certain Nora had died inside of me. Weeping softly into the pillow, I hugged my arms tightly around my middle. The weight of the last eight months of grief that I believed had been lifted away fell back upon me again, like second-story bricks crumbling into the basement of a building, where I was being buried once more by bereavement.

I thought getting pregnant again would fix parts of my grief, not bring it back to bubble up. It was barely day one of this possible pregnancy, and I was already in disbelief about its outcome.

How was I supposed to be pregnant for nine more months?

"Please stay," I whispered my wish out loud with my arms wrapped around my waist. The first wish of three I would make over the next nine months, where I hoped some make-believe genie would grant them.

chapter 25

TOO BEAUTIFUL
FOR EARTH

"Don't forget to grab Nora," I shouted to Nick in the hallway while packing our suitcase after work in late August.
The next day we were heading four hours north to Lake Superior, where we planned on spreading part of Nora's ashes. We had
waited until summer to give her back to Mother Earth when it
was warmer.

"We need to take a screwdriver with us to open her urn. I'll
run down to the basement to get one. Can you pack her ashes?"
Nick asked, as I finished folding a T-shirt and placed it in our
shared suitcase.

"Sure," I replied, before making my way to her nursery.

Opening the door to her room, the summer's sunlight shone
through the window. I had forgotten how different the sparse space
looked compared to last December. On that August afternoon,
the nursery looked more like a Pottery Barn showroom than an
actual room ready for a baby. The prepped bassinet and changing
table full of baby powder scented wipes were no longer there. The
dresser that once had bottles and a breast pump upon it was dusty,
while the crib I tried not to look at stood untouched. The white
floor-to-ceiling tree trunk decals with birds placed flying freely

reminded me of the black birds at Faith's Lodge and the three sparrows during the half-marathon . . . they reminded me of Nora flying free and away from us. The birch trees were the centerpiece of her nursery, planned around Dr. Seuss's *The Lorax* and his saying, "I speak for the trees," but it was the birds that had stayed with me . . . that made me think of her.

Picking up Nora's urn off her dresser, a single square appeared in the thick layer of lint lingering behind, similar to the shapes left in the scrapes of dough after cutting out cookies. I spotted my meditation cushion on the floor where my mother's rocking chair used to be.

When had I last meditated after focusing on my Grief Project's healing technique of "Sitting with Grief" in April? My thoughts flashed to the vision of Nora at age four, walking and playing on the beach with me. Rays of summer sunlight sparkled in the puddles of water that filled my eyes at the memory. All of me ached for her still, like it did then. Closing the door to Nora's nursery, I walked back to my room, and placed her urn in my suitcase for tomorrow's trip.

"I found the screwdriver," Nick said, entering the bedroom with it held up in his hand. Together we looked down at our child's ashes, peculiarly packed snugly between our T-shirts and shorts. Gibran's poem filled my mind once more. "You may house their bodies but not their souls."

The next day, we arrived at Bluefin Bay, the resort we had stayed at a little over two years before on our honeymoon. Nick placed Nora's urn on the nightstand next to him before going to bed.

We rose with the sun the next morning in hopes of finding the right place to put Nora to rest. In an airless and muggy Saturday afternoon, after a cool breezy morning of taking different hikes to different trails and beaches that didn't seem quite right, we found a tucked-away path hidden among the dense trees. Nick and I hiked until we came to an incline showing the way to the top of Carlton Peak, a small overlook within the Sawtooth Mountains.

Along the hike, we passed beautiful purple periwinkle wild-flowers that grew out of broken rocks and desolate terrain. Butterflies fluttered and flitted. The serenity of the surround-ings seemed surreal—almost enchanted. So peaceful and so *right*! As Nick and I climbed each large stone that led upward, we both knew this was the place.

"This trail is different," he said.

I smiled and nodded. There was a heart-shaped rock in my path like the ones we had painted at Faith's Lodge. At first, I saw just one. But then there were more. These heart stones were embedded in the trail, calling us toward the top. Dare I say, it was her guiding us to where she wanted to be.

When we reached the peak, we stood on massive boulders and walked through the trees that still managed to grow in their large cracks of soil before it turned to stone. Just past the last line of foliage, there was a clearing with an amazing view. We saw for miles the sprawling white pine and birch-wooded forest hundreds of feet below that butted up next to the never-ending Lake Superior. It was spiritual. It was perfect. It was here that we knew Nora would find her forever home.

Throughout the hike, Nick had been carrying Nora with care in his cargo pants pocket, like I imagined he would have in a hik-ing backpack if she were alive. I breathed in the beauty as Nick scouted the top terrain. Mother Nature's mixed smell of pine trees and fresh air made me realize that even though she had taken Nora away from me, it was within her hands of sky, sunlight, and soil where I found the most peace. Mother Nature was my goddess of life and death. In Hindu, they have a name for her—Goddess Kali—a figure of motherly love, both creator and destroyer of all things. Life and death being two different sides of the same coin she flipped in the air. Her game of chance, not a plan, we all played. Death was just the price we paid for life.

Still pacing back and forth, Nick continued to search the slate while scanning the view.

"This is *it!*" Nick yelled. He reached into his pocket and pulled out a clear plastic bag with gray grit inside. Gently, and with a tender touch, he opened it. Streaks formed wet streams down his face from under his sunglasses at the sight of his daughter in the shape of ash.

"Do you want to go first?" Nick asked, walking back from the ledge and toward me. I waited by a pine sapling struggling success-fully to stem from soil sprinkled in the cracks of the solid boulder I sat upon. The tree growing out of the wound in the rock reminded me of the Rumi poem I had read early in the month for August's Grief Project healing technique of "Reading Spiritual Books." It read, "The wound is the place where the light enters you."

Like the sapling, we, too, were trying to sprout from that same deep place of darkness. We would each take a turn holding Nora one last time by ourselves and then together. Nick went first. Perched by the edge, he reached into the bag and scooped up rem-nants of Nora's body, now tiny particles, that rested in his palm. He whispered words to her that I would never know before he released her onto the wind.

Then it was my turn. Nick carefully poured Nora's ashes into my cupped hand. Wrapping my fingers around her dusty form, I dug my nails into the skin of my palm, unsure if I wanted to let her leave. Pieces of her I created and never wanted to see set-tled like sand between my fingertips. My briefly beautiful baby now consisted of tiny chips of bones mixed with what looked like ground-up gravel and felt smooth against my skin. Lifting her to the wind and before blowing her away, I whispered, "Thank you for making me a mom." Scared, I hesitated for a moment. But I knew I would never be able to hold her in the form I'd hoped, so I gave her ashes one last kiss and released her onto the wind. A puff of her dust hung in the air, falling like fog over the tops of the trees. She moved from one mother's arms to another as she drifted down into Mother Nature's keeping.

With my hands still gray, like the chimney sweeper's in *Mary Poppins*, a smile rose on my face while examining the parts of Nora that had remained in the crevices of my hand. Nick joined me.

"Let's be together one last time as a family," he said, before placing another small amount of ash back into the still smoky-gray patch in the center of my palm.

Closing his hand around mine, Nick wept. "We will always love you," he promised.

And then we let her go. Once again onto the wind she sailed, and I cried, falling into Nick's arms under the warm summer sun.

When the sobs finally settled into sniffles, I turned my face up to Nick's, still partly nuzzled under his arm. "Do you think we will get to keep this baby?"

Nick placed one hand on my small, barely-there bump, and said, "I hope so."

chapter 26

THE DEFINITION
OF INSANITY

In early September, I sat in the lobby of my doctor's office with a clipboard. My pregnancy test had turned positive four weeks prior, and I scheduled an appointment with my primary provider, unable to get in with my gynecologist. I read over the questionnaire on the clipboard. *How many times in the past two weeks have you been feeling down, depressed, or hopeless?*

I wasn't sure how to answer. Wasn't it normal for someone in grief to have these emotions? Should I have been done with my mourning by then, as it had been nine months since she was gone, just as long as she had been here?

There is no time limit on grief, my therapist and psychology books told me, but I sometimes wondered if society thought otherwise. Even I thought that once we spread Nora's ashes my mourning would have magically lightened a little.

Grief, I'd been learning, was more like a spiral than a linear line.

"For in grief nothing 'stays put,'" C.S. Lewis wrote in *A Grief Observed*. "One keeps on emerging from a phase, but it always recurs."

A month ago, I would have thought grief's spirals were slowing as the crying fits in the car, shower, or behind the office door had subsided somewhat. But without warning they often resurfaced, especially when I saw another baby. It's why I made sure to sit with my back turned to the newborn snuggled into her mother's arms in the waiting room.

Even though I had learned grief was just love longing for its beloved—my keepsake for loving—I still wanted this incessant circling to stop. But instead, the spiraling had sped up since finding out I was pregnant again, causing a weird sense of déjà vu. Last year, I was sitting in this same waiting room, then five months pregnant, now I was maybe five weeks.

How often have you felt that you were a failure, having let yourself or your family down? Tapping my pen against the clipboard, I contemplated how to answer. Since getting a positive plus sign on my pee stick, I had fallen back into feeling like my body would fail me once more. I held my breath every time I went to the bathroom, afraid when pulling down my pants I would find a red stain on the lining of my underwear, or drops of blood that would turn the toilet bowl water a crimson color. It was impossible to believe my body would be able to protect life a second time around, and I was back to thinking that even though she didn't want to, Ms. Body still failed my first baby.

How difficult has it been for you to take part in daily life? My options were: *not difficult at all; somewhat difficult; very difficult; or extremely difficult.* I looked out the waiting room window as I thought. It was the beginning of September and the leaves on the trees hinted at the maroons and golds they would soon become.

If grief was like a spiral, similar to a snail shell with the Fibonacci sequence—a kind of growth pattern found in nature—then maybe I would grow from this grief, too. For like the succulent on the office assistant's desk, the sunflower in the autumn wreath on the nurse's station door, and my own thumbprint, all shared the same sequence. The building blocks of being—DNA, hurricanes, and galaxies—all possessed this pattern of growth, too. Mathematicians and scientists referred to it as the code of life. Even my fetus had taken on a similar shape, according to my pregnancy app. It was fascinating how death left behind a natural process found in nature for the bereaved to grieve that was the same in shape to the structure that babies took to form.

Noticing the *Pregnancy and Newborn* magazine on the side table next to me, I grimaced at the blooming belly bursting from its cover. Any thought of growing from grief vanished as I envied the pregnant woman who had her hands happily wrapped around her bump, seemingly unaware of the dangers that can lie inside one's own womb.

Returning to the questionnaire, I concluded that everything wasn't *extremely difficult* anymore but being pregnant again wasn't making things any easier. It made me feel kind of insane. Being pregnant after losing a child felt like the definition of insanity. I was doing the exact same thing but expecting a different result. I checked the box next to *very difficult* because feeling anxious all the time wasn't going in the direction of feeling all right.

Reviewing my score on the assessment, one would assume I was deeply depressed. But I didn't feel depressed. To me, my symptoms were just a normal response of a human trying to heal from heartbreak.

Where grief and depression overlapped or didn't was a hot debate between the mental health and grief community, arguing over what was considered mourning versus melancholy and if it should be diagnosed. Early after Nora's death, I know I felt dead inside. But I never really wanted to die. Grief intuitively felt like a natural, healthy, and normal process of sadness needed for healing after the death of a loved one.

In big letters across the bottom of the page by my final score, I wrote, "My daughter was stillborn. I'm not depressed, I'm still grieving." I underlined, underlined, and circled it.

"Lindsey Henke," The nurse called my name.

"Congratulations!" said the middle-aged doctor, whose brown hair brushed the top of her white lab coat. "The test results indicate you're about six weeks pregnant," she added cheerfully. She sat next to me on her sliding stool. The exam room had the familiar, and since Nora's stillbirth, frightening smell of antiseptic.

I blinked blankly back at this woman wearing glasses and a grin, hoping she wouldn't notice how my face morphed into a confused contortion in response to her excitement. I thought she would remember that pregnancy for me wasn't guaranteed and deliver the news with less cheer.

"Thanks," I mumbled, as she finished typing a note on her computer. I wasn't sure how I wanted my perky provider to respond, but her hopeful response made my stomach feel queasy. I was no longer willing to let hope hold the one egg I had in my basket.

I spent the rest of the month of September focused on blogging. My Grief Project was "Using Acts of Kindness to Heal," and I challenged myself to do thirty acts of kindness in thirty days in honor of Nora. I posted each deed done with a picture to my Instagram account. Other bereaved moms even did some of their own in honor of Nora, too. Tiffany, my first bereaved mom friend, who's redheaded baby boy was also born sleeping on his due date, sent me a poem in the mail. Another grieving mother of two miscarried babies took pictures of flowers and made memes out of Nora's name, with notes that said, "Nora was thinking of you."

A mother who lost her little Liam to preterm labor tipped the barista extra when paying for her cup of coffee, leaving a

THE DEFINITION OF INSANITY

Post-it note stating the good deed was done in honor of a little girl named Nora, no longer with us. Like in the early days right after Nora died when Nick and I were being cared for and carried by the unconditional love of family and friends, I again was kept afloat by the sisterhood of loss that circled me in my online world. Other bereaved moms were the best friends you never hoped to have.

Apathy about my current pregnancy settled into my soul as I went through the motions of caring for a blooming baby in my belly but held no affinity for it. I obsessed everyday about all the ways this baby might die—miscarriage from a blighted ovum, an ectopic pregnancy, or a possible chromosomal defect. At the same time, I acted like my baby might live. I gave up alcohol and ate the right foods while staying away from the supposedly wrong ones. I detached rather than attached because I couldn't take the insanity that came from constantly fearing this baby might die, too.

This dissonance only became stronger when morning sickness began. It reminded me that I was once again pregnant with a child I believed would die, while at the same time the waves of nausea and the taste of bile that built in the back of my throat comforted me in knowing that the maybe-baby inside of me was still a possibility. The feeling of incongruence only grew with the weeks that slowly pushed out my waistband.

Around week ten as the weather got cooler, Nick and I made chocolate chip cookies to keep us warm and ate them soon after baking. The cookies were still soft in the middle, and I called my mother sobbing, worried that listeria, salmonella, or my most feared bacteria, *E. coli*— the one that killed Nora—lurked inside the squishy, barely baked dough.

I had already told my parents hesitantly that we were pregnant the week before over the phone.

Dad replied, "Keep us posted." A lack of hope conveyed across the line. There were no excited words of, "We're going to be grandparents!" like the first time.

"If I get food poisoning, will I kill the baby again?" I cried into the phone's speaker to my mom. I was freaking out in our bedroom with the door closed, trying to hide my paranoia from Nick. For twenty minutes, my mother listened patiently as she tried calming me down.

But the anxiety didn't end there. I would politely ask Subway sandwich makers to change their gloves before they built my sub and ordered only a veggie sandwich with cheese to avoid lunch meat. In the breakroom at work, I attempted to nuke the neuroticism out of my mind by microwaving my meal for thirty seconds, trying to kill any listeria that lingered behind, wilting the spinach, pickles, and tomatoes between the then-warm and soggy sandwich bread in the process. I sacrificed the enjoyable taste of food for the calmness of my conscience.

I also called my doctor's office nurse line no less than twice a week regarding foods consumed. I asked my new best friend, Nurse Jessy, strange questions like, "Is it okay that I ate pepperoni on pizza that didn't seem totally cooked all the way through?" or "Should I be tested for listeria because I ate a salad with romaine lettuce recently recalled in a faraway state?"

Nurse Jessy thankfully attended to my every concern and never talked to me like the Looney Tune I saw myself becoming.

Anna didn't call me crazy, either. She referred to these incidents and all others as health anxiety. I called it PTSD from the suddenness of Nora's death. To be fair, Anna knew it was probably both. But after Nora died, the combination of previous health anxiety and the trauma of losing a baby inside my body caused me to border on the brink of paranoia, believing once again in superstitions like jinxing this pregnancy by counting my one egg before it hatched.

Fearing failure again, when I was around eleven weeks along, I pushed Nick's hand away from my belly, as he tried to pat my petite paunch.

"I'm just kind of pregnant," I reminded him. We stood in front of the stove, moving our morning meal of scrambled eggs around the frying pan with a spatula.

"You can't be sort of pregnant. You either are or are not," he retorted in response to my rejection, repeating my gynecologist's previous words. But I would argue with both. For what was I then in the last hours of pregnancy with Nora when there was the body of a baby inside of me but there was no being in that body? Wouldn't that fall into the category of kind of pregnant?

"I'm getting the feeling Nick wants to be more involved in this pregnancy," I told Anna in therapy later that week. We met in her new space located in an office park complex. Her recently purchased, dusty-gray couch had less give in its cushion. I propped myself up against the bright yellow pillows spritzed with the lavender essential oil from the bottle on the coffee table between us.

"Is that a bad thing?" she asked as she sat cross-legged in her new therapist chair, an orange-and-yellow retro thrift store find, with her new pixie haircut and a newly nude ring finger that once wore a wedding band.

I pretended to be distracted by the overwhelming newness of the place to delay my answer. A large white IKEA bookshelf bragged more brashly in the stark space while frames waited for prints propped up against the wall and the commercial carpet. "This past weekend he tried to touch my tummy, and I didn't like it. People don't understand. Even Nick doesn't. It's not like last time where we said 'when' the baby gets here. Now it's 'if' the baby lives. Everything's different this time because of what happened last time. Maybe I sound crazy? I know I feel crazy."

"You're not crazy, and you don't sound crazy." Softening her eyes, Anna continued. "You're just trying to protect yourself from getting hurt. It even has a term. It's called emotional cushioning and is common in moms pregnant again after a previous pregnancy loss. While at the same time you're trying to protect this as you say, maybe-baby, from harm, too." She nodded toward my middle. "But do you remember Nick had said he felt like he was waiting to be a dad?"

I tried recalling the conversations she referenced, but it took place in her old office when I was in the early days of my mourning, clouded in grief.

"Birth was the event that would make him a father," she said. "You were already a mom, having nine months of mothering Nora during pregnancy. Nick was waiting those nine months for her birth to become Nora's dad."

When Anna explained this to me, I realized how unique Nora's and my relationship really was, one soul that only really knew one other. I was the only person on earth that she had touched, and the only one who had held her when she was alive. The only one that truly knew her, as much as she was ever to be known. And she only knew me. Could mothers and their stillborn babies be soulmates or twin flames? My face flushed with the familiar feeling of tears about to fall, not only because Anna's explanation illustrated the profound binding between Nora's being and mine, but also because it made Nick's grief sadder to me.

Nick longed for an early connection with this baby because he had so little with Nora. He thought he would have time to get to know Nora once she was here. Now, he wanted to make up for this regret by being more involved with this baby.

"Is that how it felt for you?" I asked Nick, that evening while standing again in front of the stove. This time we made stir fry instead of scrambled eggs.

"Yeah," he replied softly.

"I'm sorry"—my lip quivered—"for pushing you away the other day. I'm just scared that this baby will die, too." I burst into tears, releasing the pressure building everywhere in my body to keep this baby alive. I knew all my neuroticisms had been illogical. This was a different pregnancy, with a different baby, with a different story, with hopefully a different ending. But this pregnancy felt like déjà vu.

Nick moved toward me. "It's going to be okay," he whispered in my ear, as I sobbed into his shoulder.

"You don't know that!" I pulled slightly away. "I told you I don't like it when you say that. The last time you said it was when the nurse left the delivery room to get the doctor right before he couldn't find Nora's heartbeat. And everything was *not* okay."

"You're right. We don't know what's going to happen," he gently reframed.

I allowed my head to fall back on his bicep, where he held me as my weeping dwindled to a wheeze. Nick's supportive embrace said without words, "I'm here. We're here together." Because really that was the only thing that could be said with certainty.

chapter 27

THE SAFE ZONE

"Life starts all over again when it gets crisp in the fall," F. Scott Fitzgerald wrote. And a new life, in the beginning of its gestation, continued blooming in my belly as October ushered in autumn. I had been pregnant for eleven weeks, almost into the supposed safe zone of the second trimester, when I dropped Nick off in downtown Minneapolis at the beginning of the Twin Cities Marathon on a cool fall morning.

"Good luck," I said, before kissing him goodbye near the starting line, knowing I wouldn't see him again until he reached the steps of Minnesota's State Capitol in Saint Paul.

While walking across the street toward the car, I thought about how we almost crossed the finish line of our previous pregnancy. It seemed absurd to me there could ever be a so-called safe zone in any pregnancy, especially this one.

Hearing the beginning notes of the national anthem play over the speakers, I searched for Nick one more time. I thought he would have been farther down the road and closer to the beginning gate, but to my surprise he stood in the same spot in the back of the line. Other runners dressed in athletic shorts and wicked tank tops under sweatshirts buzzed around him, jogged toward the crowded start, said goodbye and good luck to their loved ones, or stretched and jumped to keep warm. But not Nick. He stood with his hat over his heart, eyes facing the flag that hung from the steel rod above the start sign.

I smiled as I watched him. A proud tear rolled from my eye and onto my chilled cheek as I witnessed Nick's dedication to his role of a soldier shine through the sea of other runners. Surprised, I caught a glimpse of his dedication to being his daughter's dad, too. There was white lettering on the back of his lime-green T-shirt he must have been wearing under his sweatshirt. The recorded crescendo of the national anthem played in the background and my smile widened into a gleeful grin as I mouthed out loud the printed words upon Nick's broad shoulders.

"Nora's Dad."

Nick was running this race for Nora. The training and hours of preparation and practice was his way to be with her, honor her, and be a father to her in his own unseen and silent way. At the marathon, he no longer had to parent his daughter only while his feet pounded the pavement. Today, he was Nora's Dad to every other runner and onlooker that he passed (or passed him) over the next twenty-one miles.

A few hours later while standing on the sideline, a woman holding a poster over the barricade shouted, "Go Team Nora!"

Nick came down the hill, picking up his pace to reach the finish line. She had read Nick's T-shirt. Nick slowed down his jog to a bouncing walk as he passed me, proudly pointing to the letters on the front of his lime-green tee.

"Go Team Nora!" I shouted this time, cheering out loud in unexpected unison with the supportive lady next to me. When hearing his daughter's name screamed excitedly across the street toward him, Nick's eyes grinned wider than his smile. He was Nora's dad for everyone at the run!

Once Nick crossed the finish line and crawled out of the

crowd, I found him with a gold finisher's medal around his neck. He huffed for air and sweat profusely but seemingly happy with his accomplishment.

"You did it!" I yelled in excitement, as I hugged him despite his sour stench.

"Yeah," he puffed and smiled as he tried breathing.

Pulling away, I said softly, "I like your shirt."

"You do?" He smiled again.

"I do," I replied with an approving grin.

Nick had successfully finished his marathon, but I still had two-thirds of what felt like a marathon pregnancy ahead of me, with my most recent EDD being calculated for April 15.

"Tax Day," is what the nurse teasingly tossed out while checking my pulse on my lunch break at a drop-in appointment. A sharp shot of lightning had ripped through my groin during a therapy session with a client, causing a nervous spiral to start.

"Probably round ligament pain," was what Nurse Jessy said over the phone when I called her from work. Her uncertain diagnosis didn't calm my undulating unease. For as my waistband grew, so did my worries. Almost thirteen weeks along, the first trimester symptoms of nausea, achy breasts, and fatigue had faded without any reassuring replacement of flutters from movements made by my maybe-baby. *Am I still pregnant if my boobs are no longer sore?* I wondered. Maybe the receding symptoms were because the baby was dead, not because I was in the presumed honeymoon period of the second trimester that happily pregnant moms on baby boards bragged about. For me, reaching this mock milestone only offered another stage of trepidation to trudge through.

My knee bounced up and down frantically under my desk like a monkey jumping on a bed. I needed to be sure this baby's heart was still beating or I wouldn't make it through the rest of the workday. I had expected to feel more anxious about being pregnant again after losing Nora, but I never thought worry would be as persistent as it was. A cramp from constipation or an ache in my side was mistaken for contractions. *Will this baby live?*

Lying on a cool, plastic-covered exam table, with the scary scent of antiseptic in the air, my middle was exposed, once again vulnerable to whatever words would shape my fate. I recalled the last time I laid in the same position. My belly was watermelon-sized instead of the small mound protruding against my midsection muscles. I barely heard the squishing sound of the blue gel out of its bottle and onto my goosebump-covered belly over my heavy heartbeat.

The nice nurse was not Nurse Jessy but an older woman with grandmotherly hands. She smiled and chatted about the weather as Minnesotans often do during moments of painful pauses in conversations. She mentioned something about it being unusually warm for October while she placed the plastic bottle the blue goo came from back on the shelf and reached for the Doppler attached to a small speaker on the wall behind me. I hadn't had a Doppler wand stroke my skin since that early morning months ago when the doctor declared Nora dead.

"I can hear your heartbeat," said the nurse unconcerned, as she turned up the speaker before she continued moving the lubricated wand from one hip bone over the bump below my belly button and across to the other.

For a moment I couldn't breathe. With my head resting on the crinkly paper-covered pillow and my legs dangling off the edge of the exam table, I closed my eyes and recited a silent prayer even though I didn't pray. *Please be there. Please be there.*

The nurse's face turned from a look of calmly carrying on casual conversation to concern. She passed the wand one more time over my middle with no reassuring noise besides static reverberating from the speakers. Then she spoke a similar sentence I had heard another nurse in my past pacify me with. "Sometimes it's hard to find the heartbeat. I'll go get the doctor." Her words confirmed the look of fear I had read on her face.

Biting the corner of my lip so hard I thought I tasted blood, I shifted my head away from the nurse's face toward the comforting blank slate of the sterile white wall. *How could this happen again?* A stream of hot tears worked their way down my cheeks and created puddle prints in the flimsy paper pillow. Closing my eyes tighter, I pleaded harder and directly to Death herself who I feared floating once more around the room. "Please don't do this to me again. Please don't take another one of my babies."

Just like last time, a doctor I had never met appeared by my side, ahead of the nervous nurse who returned with a portable ultrasound. The overhead lights were switched off, allowing me to focus on the doctor's eyes and her carefully controlled features, lit by the eerie bluish glow of the screen. Watching the event unfold, I didn't speak or dare ask if everything was okay. I knew she didn't yet know.

Doing a sort of sit-up onto my elbows, I brought my head and shoulders off the table while keeping my stomach still, which gave me the view I needed to stare at the doctor's face where I continued to search for familiar clues of safety or seriousness. She wasn't my doctor, but she must have looked at my chart for she kept the ultrasound screen toward her and away from me as her hand moved across my barely bulging bump. Then I noticed her larger one poking out from her lab coat. This doctor was pregnant herself, probably seven months along I estimated. *Of course, fate would fuck me in this way again,* I thought, as the seriousness of her stoic face refused to soften. Not being able to watch this performance play out a second time, I allowed my shoulders to fall back onto the exam table, where the paper crunched beneath my back. I squeezed my eyes sharply shut, like shutters blocking out the sun.

"There!" The doctor almost shouted. "There's your baby," she said, pointing at the screen. The satisfied smile she made toward the monitor moved to meet my ghostly gaze. "At this stage they're still tiny, about the size of a lime, and move around a lot. That's why they're sometimes hard to find." She sounded almost as relieved as I was. "Your baby looks great."

"Is the baby, okay?" I asked, still shaking.

"As far as I can tell, yes," she nodded and returned her stare to the screen to double-check her assessment. "Baby has a heart rate of 156 beats per minute, which is completely normal for this stage of the pregnancy." Turning the sound up on the speakers, she moved the monitor toward me. There in black-and-white was a little bean that resembled a baby bouncing around the bubble inside my belly. A *flub, flub, flub,* pulsated from the playback of the recorded footage.

My arms and legs shivered. The adrenaline from fear was working its way out of my system. The doctor said the baby and pregnancy were *normal,* even though nothing felt normal anymore.

"I can't imagine how hard this is for you."

I remained muted, only being able to nod.

"We are here for whatever you need."

I blinked back tears. *I need it to be Tax Day,* I thought, as I left the exam room and headed to my car. I laid my head on the steering wheel, letting streams of tears flow as fast as my racing heartbeat. We had reached the so-called safe zone in pregnancy, but nothing seemed safe. Nothing would until I crossed the finish line of this pregnancy holding a breathing baby in my arms. Placing my palm on top of my middle protruding from my skinny jeans that I could no longer button, I softly whispered, "Please stay."

chapter 28

ANNOUNCING BEING KNOCKED UP

The Doppler disaster of an appointment only confirmed our previously made plans of waiting to publicly announce this pregnancy. By mid-October, we were fourteen weeks along and like the pumpkins on our porch surrounded by the unpleasant scent of decaying leaves, I, too, was round in the middle, but we hadn't yet shared our secret on social media, still unsure when the right time to tell the world would be. And because of this, other things waited as well, including weekly bump pictures or purchasing any item for the maybe-baby. Both acts of hope we happily embraced once starting the second trimester with Nora, we now winced away from.

Even with a blooming belly, I continued believing death could be the only outcome of birth and refused to buy maternity attire. While shopping at Target, I avoided the baby and maternity aisles. I never considered wearing the old pregnancy clothes I had boxed away in the back of my closet, fearing if I put on an outfit I once wore with a failed pregnancy, it would be tempting another sad fate.

However, this avoidance tactic was becoming difficult to execute at the office. At fifteen weeks pregnant, those who saw me every day had likely noticed the shift in my wardrobe from wearing fitted tops and sleek slacks to flowy bum-covering blouses and stretchy leggings. The oversized outfits may have been successful at hiding my bump, but I could no longer handle the pressure that came with pretending this pregnancy wasn't present.

"I need help," I told Bridget, my new supervisor, after taking a seat on her pillow-filled couch. My previous supervisor had left for a new job in the last month, and I turned to my current boss for advice.

Bridget was a warm, round woman in her late forties, with short spiky gray hair, a nose ring, and a spunky personality to match. In private company she described herself as an actual witch, alluding to her Wiccan ways by sprinkling trinkets throughout her office. A dark oblong mystical mask hung on the wall by her window, a wooden magical wand with a yellow star on top peeked out from her pen jar, and I nervously fidgeted with the colorful crystals on the end table. She was a brilliant therapist and mentor, mostly because she brought a little bit of her magic into her work. If I unfairly labeled my previous supervisor as a wicked witch, Bridget became my dressed-in-all-black Glinda. I really did wish, like Dorothy, that I could click my heels together, hunker down, and hide for the rest of this pregnancy.

"I've never done this before," I continued, avoiding Bridget's eyes by rolling one of her clear crystal rocks through my fingers, "but I need to transfer a client." When my client started shaking in session, I trembled inside. Her trauma was different from mine but triggered my own well of wounds. "Her emotions seemed to seep into me instead of me being able to hold them." I had lost the capacity to be a container for clients' feelings because my own nervous energy was unraveling on the floor like a ball of yarn a kitten was trying to catch.

"Are you sure, Lindsey?" She tilted her head to the side and her short hair with spiked gray tips swayed, too. "This doesn't seem like you. I mean, I will if you want. It's just that you've been through so much and have managed to work quite well with clients, considering." Blinking behind her bookworm eyeglasses resting on the tip of her nose, she asked, "Is there something I'm missing?"

"I'm pregnant!" I hoped blurting out the phrase would have the same effect as tearing off a Band-Aid and getting the uncomfortable experience over with quickly.

Bridget nodded without a well-meaning "Congrats!" or a concerned, "How are you doing?" Instead, her face stayed softly solid and welcoming as she said, "Ah, I understand. This is making more sense now."

"Well, I'm glad you understand," I said sarcastically, while shaking my head, "because I don't. All I know is everything has become more overwhelming."

Bridget's thin eyebrows drew together as she listened.

"Since Nora died, suffering I never noticed before now seems to be everywhere. It's like I *feel* all the pain on the planet at once. Being pregnant again has made it worse, suddenly dissolving any boundary I once held between me and the outside world that was protecting me from its brutality. On top of all of that, I'm confused as to how to grieve a dead child and also feel fleeting moments of joy at the potential of a new one." I let out a large sigh and admitted, "It's just so exhausting and confusing having to feel an overwhelming sense of sadness, the possibility of hope, and hormones all at once."

A smile grew on Bridget's face before she slapped her hands onto her knees. "That's the beauty of being human, Lindsey!"

"What?" I questioned. Confused and a little concerned, I thought maybe my Glinda wouldn't be able to point me in the direction of a yellow brick road that led to a wizard who would ease my worries.

Bridget held out one hand to the left and the other to the right. "You get to feel both happy and sad at once." She finished her sentence by clasping her hands together in front of her. "Isn't that lovely?" Her sparkling eyes softened into a state of knowing wisdom acquired through one's own experience. "You've been broken open by motherhood, and now it's made you aware of all the beauty and cruelty in the world."

I pursed my lips together and digested Bridget's insights. She had explained how to hold everything I had been experiencing over the last year with the singular use of one word: *and*. It linked both the beautiful and the brutal without taking away meaning from the other, not having to choose between grief or joy. Bridget was giving me permission to be both grateful for this new baby *and* still grieve Nora. I didn't need to pick a side; I could embrace them both. I could be true to my second Grief Commandment: sadness *and* happiness could both live within grief.

"Yeah," I whispered with a nod. "It's kind of like how in grief there is still so much beauty, and really in death, too," I said, remembering how I still loved Nora in her decaying form. I contemplated who I was before Nora died compared to who I had become in the aftermath of her death. "Now I cry at things I never did before. Like TV commercials, and I'm not just talking about the desperately depressing dog commercials with their sad puppy eyes behind bars. You know the one?"

"I do." Bridget chuckled at my attempt at humor.

"But the banal ones, too, where the underdogs win the game, *and* this also means that I feel like I'm being stabbed in the heart when my clients tell me their own trauma. I don't understand the injustice. Why do some get so much pain and others so little? I can't make sense of all the cruelty in the world."

"Then don't," Bridget said matter-of-factly, as she leaned back confidently in her maroon armchair, "because you can't." Her abrupt tone then transitioned to softness, "Just remember that your heart can hold both experiences of love and loss at once. It's the beauty of being human." She winked as she shared her last tidbit of wisdom. "It's also the secret to being a mother."

Warm relief washed over me. Bridget's willingness to witness my different forms of motherhood was magical to me. She really was my Glinda, waving her magic wand over my ruby slippers of grief and joy to reveal I had the power of "and" inside of me. She challenged me to give myself permission to love both Nora *and* this new baby growing in my belly.

Just like Glinda, she left the decision for me to make.

Later that week, close to midnight, Nick slept next to me while I scrolled through Instagram and saw a photo in my feed from *Pregnancy & Newborn Magazine,* seeking applications for their next *Knocked Up Blogger.* The position description explained they were looking for a pregnant person to write weekly about their nine-month journey toward parenthood for the online publication of their magazine.

Intrigued, I opened a blank email on my phone and quickly crafted a proposal as to why they should pick me. I included the black-and-white photos of Nick and I holding Nora along with a selfie I had taken in the mirror with a positive pregnancy test.

Since the moment I threw that pregnancy test in the trash, I wondered when the right time would be to share the news with those who followed my blog. For the past three months, I had continued writing about my grief, ensuring I had completed my Grief Project for the year, but I hadn't mentioned being pregnant again. Instead, I focused on October's healing technique of "Healing Through the Arts," creating bereaved parent playlists and capturing grief in photographs. But I was barely able to post the few articles I had written. Constant fears about this pregnancy left little room to focus on writing. Nick and I had recently discussed sharing the news once I was sixteen weeks pregnant, which was four weeks farther into pregnancy than last time. If I was eventually going to write about the challenges of pregnancy after loss on my blog, then why not share my struggles with a wider audience?

I hovered the arrow over the blue send button containing my proposal's rough draft and clicked my finger on the touchpad. I sent it off to my sister, and then I sent her a text.

I sent you an email. Read it. Then tell me what you think?

Kristi, a night owl like myself, called within seconds.

"You're going to apply, right?" were the first words she cheered on the other end of the line. "You must send this. Your email is amazing!"

One cupped hand covered my whisper into the receiver. "You think so?"

"Yes. I'll look it over again in the morning and make a few edits. Then you should send it to them ASAP." Her excitement made me excited for the first time in a long time. Then she paused. "But are you ready to be this public about your pregnancy? You haven't told anyone else outside the immediate family." Kristi sighed. "I mean Lindsey, when are you going to get excited about being pregnant again?"

Kristi didn't understand that another pregnancy didn't fix my sorrow. I knew most well-meaning family and friends may have secretly hoped this to be true. I even foolishly thought my grief would get easier if we got a positive pregnancy test but being pregnant after losing a baby didn't take away the pain of missing the one who died.

My frustration with Kristi had faded since that conversation. My sister had been more supportive in my grief than anyone else. Not having children, her dedication to loving a niece she would never know amazed me. "I'm scared. I know my thoughts aren't logical, but I fear that the moment we tell others, something horrible will happen again and we'll have to un-tell everyone, just like last time. If I put this pregnancy out there, it becomes true, and once it becomes true, I'll have something to lose again."

Silence was the only sound on the other end of the receiver until I heard Kristi say, "That makes sense. But you're still going to apply for the writing gig, right?"

With the glimmer of excitement I briefly experienced at my sister's excitement, I knew my answer had to be yes. Besides, they probably wouldn't pick my story. It seemed too sad to share in a mainstream pregnancy magazine. New parents were already on edge about what could go wrong with their baby. I couldn't imagine the editors would want to risk bringing on a blogger who was an example of a pregnant parent's worst nightmare come true.

"Yes," I reassured my sister through the speaker, "I'll apply. It's not like I really have a chance."

"Well, if you don't try, you'll never know," Kristi said.

chapter 29

OTHER PEOPLE'S PREGNANCIES

While waiting to hear from the magazine, I attended routine doctor's appointments.

"All of your results look great!" Dr. Hayes said, when I was sixteen weeks pregnant, in reference to the noninvasive prenatal testing we had done. Relieved, I let out a long exhale and stood up to leave when Dr. Hayes continued, "I think it's time we talk about your birth plan."

"It's a little early to discuss that, isn't it?" I was afraid I wouldn't make it to next week let alone week thirty-seven, when we were planning on having a C-section. We had decided to deliver early because stillbirth rates rise for every pregnant person starting at thirty-seven weeks, albeit a minuscule increase. We settled on a cesarean, not because of the previous stillbirth, but because of shoulder dystocia Nora had at birth. It had a chance of recurring in future pregnancies. "So, what has changed?"

"Everything is still the same," she said with her cool and calm smile she always carried on her round face speckled with freckles. "The one thing different is that you and I have the same due date." She glanced at her still-small stomach covered by her white coat.

"Oh," tumbled out of my mouth that stayed open. I left off

the *Dear God! You're pregnant!* part and instead, coughed out, "Congrats."

"Thank you," she replied and politely turned the conversation back to me. "Since we're delivering you three weeks early, there shouldn't be a problem. I'll still be able to do the surgery." She continued to speak about birth logistics, but I no longer heard her. My mind wandered to all the other happily pregnant people who kept popping up in my life, and I added Dr. Hayes to the list.

Since losing Nora, a handful of old high school friends had shown up in my Facebook feed announcing their pregnancies.

"It's a girl," one acquaintance's post boasted in an image of her and her husband kissing as she held an ultrasound photo in front of her blooming bump. Then a coworker, who I facilitated a therapy group with, had just found out she was pregnant and talked incessantly about it.

Even being pregnant again myself, I still held a visceral disdain for other people's pregnancies because it seemed mine with Nora didn't count in their conversations. Pregnant people would shift uncomfortably in their seats when I tried to share innocuous memories from my nine months with Nora. My silence in these conversations seemed to be the response people preferred, making me lose not just Nora but the time we had spent together.

On break from teaching a group of clients coping skills to stay sober, my fellow therapist cornered me and chatted about her hopes of birthing her currently blueberry-sized baby at home and how her husband planned to catch their not-yet newborn. Needing to escape from the conversation, I excused myself, saying something about having to use the restroom, and darted into my office. I collapsed into my desk chair with a sigh of relief that I no longer had to pretend to care about my colleague's pregnancy. There was a new email from *Pregnancy & Newborn Magazine* in my inbox.

My heart pounded with anticipation, but I tried not to get my hopes up. Bracing for rejection, I moved my cursor over the bolded unopened email and clicked on it to view their reply.

"We are so sorry for your loss and would like to invite you to write weekly about your current pregnancy for *Pregnancy & Newborn Magazine.*" I leaned in closer to the screen, astonished. I reread the email three more times, just to be sure they really had chosen me.

After the group ended that night, I ran to the car and dialed Nick's number on my drive home from work.

"That's awesome, Lindsey! I'm so proud of you!"

My stomach did a somersault at his excitement, unsure if it was my own enthusiasm or this baby's first flutter. "Should I accept it?" I said into the speaker.

Nick's voice reverberated off the car's windows in response, "Yes. It's what you wanted, right? To raise awareness about what it's like to lose a baby?"

"But—" I gulped down air, "what if by sharing we are pregnant again, I'll jinx it?"

I heard Nick huff with frustration. "It doesn't work that way. You know that. Besides, we lived through it before, and we could survive it again . . . if we had too."

"Yes." I nodded my head even though Nick couldn't see me. "So, we're doing this?" I asked. I pulled into our driveway and pressed the garage door opener, hearing the murmur of its motor clatter.

"*You're* doing this!" he answered.

chapter 30

A SIBLING,
NOT A REPLACEMENT

"Do you want to know the sex of the baby?" the sonographer asked while moving a wand wet with blue gel over my belly. It was the Monday before Thanksgiving when Nick and I found ourselves once again in a darkened cave-like ultrasound room, wondering what form our future family would take.

In the last month before then, my first *Knocked Up Blogger* post had been published on *Pregnancy & Newborn's* online magazine, and it received a warm and loving response from the loss community, our family, and friends. In the picture of the post, shared the week before Halloween, Nick and I had dressed in black T-shirts with white bones while a waving little skeleton baby rested on my bump. We announced to the world we were pregnant again. Even Georgie was in the photo, chewing on a rawhide too large for his tiny mouth.

"Holding on to hope for you," a friend wrote in the comments section under the post I shared on Facebook, when at times this seemed impossible for Nick and me to do.

My mother, unimpressed with the title of my new writing position said, "You know, 'knocked up' wasn't such an endearing term when I was young." She implied my blog title was a pejorative term for a sixteen-year-old who was unexpectedly pregnant. Unlike me, a woman who had plotted her period on an app, peed on ovulation sticks, and prearranged intercourse for the last eight months, basically begging Mother Nature for another baby.

Nick and I watched that begged-for-baby bounce around the inside of my belly on a black-and-white screen at our mid-pregnancy anatomy scan. Where the sonographer, like a modern-day mystic looking into her crystal ball, once again asked if we wanted to know the sex of this baby.

Nick and I had agreed that all we wanted was a healthy baby but had different hopes for its assigned sex. Nick wanted another girl. He'd told me so a few weeks before while I laid with my back against his breastbone with his arms wrapped around my mounting middle as we watched television. "I kind of hope it's a girl," he replied after I had asked him the question the sonographer had just asked us. "I know it sounds crazy, but maybe . . ." Rubbing his thumb and fingers back and forth over my belly he spoke softly. "If it's a girl, it would be like Nora is coming back to us in a way. I know we can't replace her, but maybe it would feel like in some way she was here."

I squeezed his torso tightly, giving him a hug to acknowledge his tenderly shared wish for similarities between the present and the past. However, I kept my secret sex preference to myself. I wanted a boy.

In the dimly-lit ultrasound room, Nick squeezed my hand with the same sense of affection I had given him the week before. I repeated one final silent wish for our second baby to be a boy, believing if this child was a different sex, then this pregnancy might have a different outcome. It was a delusion I hoped to hold on to as I white-knuckled through the rest of this pregnancy.

Nick's eyes told me, without words, that he was ready to know. Nodding an affirmative toward the twenty-something technician wearing blue scrubs we uttered once more in unison, "Yes."

"It's a girl!"

The sonographer's happy exclamation echoed in my ears as my body went numb, flooding with fear at the similarities between this pregnancy and my past one. I felt like Dorothy waking up from her time in Oz, where she tells Auntie Em some of it wasn't good but most of it was wonderful.

Tears shimmered in Nick's eyes with his wish fulfilled. I smiled at him under the moonlight glow of the ultrasound screen, happy for him that his hope for a second chance at raising a daughter could possibly come true. I silently cursed the cosmos for this déjà vu pregnancy, having been here before, only fifteen months ago.

Why this baby and not Nora? I would mumble throughout the days during the weeks that followed the scan in hopes that the Universe, Mother Nature, or a God would respond. "Someone answer me," my mind would demand, before falling asleep at night, ruminating about what to write that the non-bereaved would actually read in my weekly blog for *Pregnancy & Newborn Magazine.* Or when seated next to Nick on the couch watching movies with full families as I typed posts about my healing technique for the month of November, "Gratitude while Grieving," that reluctantly pushed me to find moments to be grateful for when I was frustrated with fate.

A reveal cake was the dessert to our Thanksgiving dinner, after a turkey-filled brunch at Nick's parents' house wedged between a high-rise railroad bridge and the Sheyenne River in the frozen fields of North Dakota. During half-time of the Packers football game, Nick's parents, aunt, uncle, sister, niece, and cousins gathered around the antique dining table, where Nick had eaten his daily dinners as a child, to watch him cut into the white iced cake.

Pink frosting peaked out from where the bread knife sliced through the middle of the fluffy white buttercream and marble. Nick's mother and his aunt Susie squealed at the sight of the sweet-scented pastel icing smeared on the side of the plate, as I'm sure they did in years past when Nick blew out the candles on his birthday cakes.

Family members clapped and cheered, "It's a girl," as loud as they did for a Packer's touchdown, while I quietly forced a smile and turned my attention to the framed black-and-white photo of Nora on the nearby end table. Next to it sat one pink wilted rose resting in a small glass vase my mother-in-law had kept from Nora's funeral, a mere two feet from where everyone had just found out Nora would have a sister. *Sisters.* The familiar word suddenly felt foreign on my tongue as I whispered it to myself again. Sisters. Who will never meet.

What if others didn't see this baby as Nora's sister? What if the excitement they exuded was because they were relieved we were getting a do-over on parenthood with this daughter as a replacement for our dead one? The replacement child syndrome was a term coined by psychologists in the 1960s for a child conceived shortly after the death of another. Psychologists were concerned they would be at risk for psychopathology if the parents had not sufficiently grieved their child that died.[1]

"Am I replacing her?" I asked Anna in session on a cold but clear November morning.

Anna, dressed in a cozy cowl neck sweater and slacks, said, "You're not replacing her. I don't believe in the idea of a replacement child. It is one of many myths about bereaved parents that we now know not to be true. Bereaved parents often make space for a baby born after the loss of another, as the sibling of their child who died. This baby is Nora's sister, not a replacement."

Sighing deeply, I settled into the couch. Over the last few days, I had accepted and surprisingly even started to get a little excited about having a second chance at raising a daughter.

"But I worry that other people will forget about her." My eyebrows drew together. "And that, maybe, I might forget about her too?"

Anna returned the question to me. "Do you think you will?"

Looking out the wide window, I pondered. Dried leaves in different shades of brown had fallen from the naked trees onto the not yet snow-covered ground, rustled in the wind. "No," I finally replied. My chin trembled. "I don't think so. I still want Nora back, and this baby, too." I avoided eye contact with Anna as shame rose within my chest for not being grateful or excited for this baby. I took a breath and placed a hand on my noticeable belly. "But maybe," I continued, lifting my eyes to meet Anna's, "I can still be the kind of mother I wanted to be with Nora to this child." Tears pricked at the back of my eyes as another admission appeared. "It feels like grief has flooded me again, bringing back all those magical thoughts that because this baby is a girl, this baby will die, too."

Anna nodded as I sniffled. "That makes sense. It's called re-grief."

"Re-what?"

"Re-grief," she repeated, while smirking at my returned attempt at humor, which I used to hide my vulnerability. "It's processing grief from a different developmental perspective than was possible earlier." Anna continued, "Once you enter a new stage of development, like becoming pregnant again, you process old information from this new perspective."

Anna's explanation made sense to me, but it still didn't help settle my soul and provide answers as to why Nora had to die, and this baby might get to live.

"Why this baby, why not you?" I cried into the steam of the shower. My moans would be muffled by the steady sound of water humming as it beat off the shower basin. Huddled naked in the corner, with my hands clasped around my shins, I heard in my head, *Mama, you get to keep this one.*

Tears mingled with beads of water. Hot misty clouds had filled the stall as I lifted my head from between my knees at what I believed to be Nora answering me. It could have been my own voice. But I didn't care. Every time during the rest of my pregnancy, when I spoke directly to Nora, a reassuring voice would always answer.

Standing up, without thought, I drew a capital N through the wetness on the glass shower door, which allowed me to see clearly through to the other side. I continued carving the letters of her name out of the dew upon the door with an "ora."

"Nora," I whispered through the heat. While I traced each letter over and over again, water from the shower drummed like raindrops against my body. I decorated her name on the glass with hearts like I used to do with my own on notepads in elementary school. Missing her more than I had in months and needing her to guide me during this pregnancy, I had unknowingly started a new ritual—etching her name on the glass every morning and night, for years to come.

chapter 31

IS THIS
YOUR FIRST?

December brought with it dying as it always does. Autumn's
beautiful changing-colored leaves had moved into the year's
final season of life and, with it, Death. Branches bald with brown-
ness covered the barren landscape hinting of a coming Midwest
winter, accompanied by a chill in the air, reminding my body of the
anniversary of Nora's death, even if my mind resisted the realization.

My birthday came two weeks before Nora's. To celebrate the
day, Nick ordered my favorite Vietnamese take-out. We ate our
meal of chicken pho with rice noodles on the couch in front of the
hot ribbons of light coming from the fireplace.

"Happy birthday!" Nick said, as he stood in front of me and
opened a small white box. He pulled out an oversized chocolate cupcake covered in green frosting and lit the single candle on top with a
long lighter he snatched from the brick mantel. "Make a wish."

Sharing a happy glance, I flashed a smile back at him, my bare
feet tucked warmly under a wool blanket. The small flame flick-
ered on top of the cupcake. The only wish I could think to make
was that thirty-one would be better than thirty.

Forming my lips into a little oval, I blew out the yellow flame,
sad to be celebrating the day without my daughter. The singular

candle wick wilted, smoldering on the cupcake as a lingering small stream of smoke hung in the air. A strange feeling of frustration mixed with forlornness found me. My stomach dropped as the truth of my single birthday candle came to light. I had grown a year older when Nora would never know age one.

Passing a fork back and forth between us, we took turns taking bites out of the moist cupcake. The new little girl that took up residence in Nora's old home flipped and flopped against my womb's walls as the sugar made its way to her banana-sized body through the umbilical cord connecting us.

Connection. Something I desperately desired with this baby but also feared. Every kick, jab, and roll grew stronger from within. The little lady pushed upon my uterus, intensifying my need to connect with her. This baby had moved away from being my maybe-baby and became baby number two. Even if birthed alive, the rest of the world would see her as our only, instead of our second. But referring to her as baby number two was a sign to me that I was starting to step away from detachment and onto the shores of hope's labile landscape.

However, hope, like fairy-tale endings, was fleeting, because something else would always happen to make me fall back into bracing myself for heartbreak. The week after my birthday, at twenty-two weeks pregnant, I asked Nick to bring me to the hospital one dark December evening after work due to a sudden onset of digestive issues.

My heart fluttered fast in my chest as I stood across from Nick in the hospital elevator. He pressed the button to floor two, where I had given birth to Nora. Bracing my back against the small space's squared wall, I clasped one arm at the elbow of my other. My insides quivered. The smell of antiseptic entered my nose. I closed my eyes to push away the fear. But behind my eyelids, I saw myself as the teacher at the end of the book *Brown Bear, Brown*

Bear What Do You See? I feared that when the elevator doors slid open, all the nurses would be looking at me, the jinxed lady who delivered a dead baby. Feeling the familiar slight stomach drop of reaching our designated floor, my eyes opened, and the grinding metal doors opened, too. Stepping off the elevator into the maternity ward, my angst was on the precipice of a panic attack as my body shivered. But to my surprise, it never came because everything about the building was different.

In the time since Nora was born, the hospital had renovated the maternity department. What was once a dingy and dreary green and cream sterile lobby was transformed into a bright and welcoming one. Orange-and-yellow floral murals hung large on freshly painted white walls, where painted, pea-green brick was once prominent upon entrance. Previously stained chairs were replaced with new, comfortable, leather couches. With the change in scenery, my sensory experiences also changed. Memories of the trauma moved out of my mind, which caused my anxiety to lighten a little, just like the walls of the hospital had.

Settling into the assessment room, a young nurse asked, "Is this your first?" as she hooked me up to the same fetal monitor that never found Nora's heartbeat.

"No." Glancing quickly at Nick, I replied, "My first baby died." Nora's anniversary would soon be upon us—next week. My body reminded me with uncomfortable digestive issues of gas and diarrhea that the day was coming, even as my brain wanted to resist its impending approach. "This is our second."

A familiar flush crept across the suddenly self-conscious nurse's face. "I'm sorry." My answer caught her off guard, instead of me being caught off guard. Usually, I struggled to find a reply that felt honest and true to both my children. People didn't understand that pregnancies were personal and shouldn't be mentioned in making superficial small talk.

The embarrassed nurse's expression softened and so did her tone. "What is the worry that brings you in?"

"Preterm labor." But this was only half true. The other half was Nora's anniversary.

Creeping closer to Christmas and to what should have been Nora's first birthday soon after, I struggled to focus. I was only able to write one blog post the last month of my Grief Project about December's healing technique of "Resting, Remembering, and Reflecting," and I really wasn't interested in reflecting.

When I reflected, I ruminated on how I once imagined Nora would have been eating a smash cake while sitting in her highchair for her first birthday, instead of being reduced to rubble remains in an urn on the unused dresser in an empty nursery. My subconscious took me back to the trauma from the year before.

But instead of admitting this to myself, I focused on the fear that at twenty-two weeks pregnant, if this baby were born alive, she likely wouldn't survive. A Dr. Google search had informed me that cramping and diarrhea could be symptoms of preterm labor. Entering each new week of pregnancy, a new way to lose this baby always accompanied it.

"Everything looks great." The doctor with tightly curled hair and a mother's weathered face reassured Nick and I after completing her exam. "Probably just an upset stomach caused by stress. After everything you've been through, it's normal to be concerned . . . and to want reassurance." Her steady gaze radiated with understanding of the unfairness of our fate. "If you need to come back twenty more times before the end of your pregnancy, you can. That's what we're here for." She touched my hand. "You're coming up on hard times. Anniversaries of losses and the holidays can be difficult for the grieving." She sympathetically smiled, and I wiped away a grateful tear.

chapter 32

CHRISTMAS
BLUES

On Christmas Eve morning, twenty-three weeks pregnant with baby number two, I ran my fingers over Nora's Santa stocking that would forever remain unfilled. It hung over the fireplace next to Nick, who gathered gifts from under the sparsely-decorated artificial table tree and placed the presents and suitcases, like jigsaw puzzle pieces, into the trunk of the car. We were headed to my parents' house for Christmas.

As the holiday approached, my body became heavier under the weight of not only the baby growing in my belly but the new mounting sorrow that the day symbolized—the beginning of the end we didn't know was upon us last year.

Staring at the Santa sock, I was reminded of the previous Christmas, when I hung Nora's expectant stocking between Nick's and mine on the mantel. Her birth was like a coveted gift I had written on my wish list nine months before. But this year, I didn't dare situate a new stocking in between Nick's and mine.

Before getting on the road, I ran upstairs to our bedroom, remembering one more thing to take along.

Standing in front of my dresser, I reached for Nora's footprint necklace. It was still suspended in the air, hanging from the wooden dowel by the oblong mirror, where I had left it and hadn't touched it since Father's Day. Holding the silver pendant between my pointer finger and thumb, I wiped away the thin layer of dust that had settled into the grooves of Nora's engraved footprint. Taking each end of the chain in one hand, I watched my reflection in the mirror as my arms floated around my neck and found each other on the other side. The cool pendant met my skin in the dip between my clavicle. Closing the clasp, it fell to the base of my neck, resting on the top bump of my spine. Inhaling deeply, my chest rose, and I closed my eyes. All was calm but nothing felt right, as the slight thrill of hope of baby number two growing in my belly was at odds with the anniversary of Nora's death nearing.

Nick and I made it through the winter wonderland that blanketed the interstate from Minneapolis to southern Wisconsin in time to spend Christmas Eve at my grandmother's house, a tradition I had done since childhood. My memories of Christmas at Grandma and Grandpa's were imprinted with the scent of cigar mingled with cut evergreens and freshly-baked sugar cookies. Presents were piled so high around a trimmed tree, they seemed to almost touch the ceiling that the treetop pressed upon, where no topper ever had room to fit. Laughter was loud during the holiday season and every year, everyone, or at least someone, always chuckled while commenting on the oversized and over-piled-with-presents Tannenbaum.

In the last few years, the magic of our childhood Christmas dwindled when Aunt Mary became sick and Grandpa's cancer diagnosis soon followed. On Christmas Eve during the illness-filled years, presents were still stacked high around the tree as we all tried pretending the holiday was merry and Death wasn't planning a visit. But the laughter was low, and sarcastic sullenness quietly suffused the once ruckus-filled room. Then with the death of both

Grandpa and Aunt Mary, Christmas seemed to have in some way died, too, along with my childhood.

Death always takes a child, I've come to believe, whether an actual child or childhood innocence.

However, this year a sense of celebration shifted into the season. The living room, once saturated with sarcasm, transformed back into the happy holiday setting of my youth. More joy than grief finally filled my grandmother, uncle, and cousin's despondent days. This newfound happiness came in the form of tiny tots named Quinn and Braxton. They chased each other around my grandmother's galley kitchen, as I leaned against her cupboards brushing crumbs from a stiff snowman sugar cookie off my baby bump covered in a turtleneck maternity sweater.

Quinn, who had just turned one, briskly walked, not waddled, past me as he gleefully giggled at his three-month younger cousin Braxton's inability to catch him. Braxton, who had been the baby in my cousin's wife's belly at Nora's funeral, was trying hard, but failed to reach Quinn, as he wobbled on all fours behind his more mobile playmate. Both boys, now more toddlers than babies, were followed by one of their respective parents as they hunched over with their protective parental arms stretched wide to catch their child from a future faceplant.

How did Quinn, a Buddha baby unable to even sit up when I last saw him nine months ago, run around my grandmother's throw rug-filled kitchen without falling? Sadly, I realized that I didn't know anything about a baby past birth. I had no real understanding of what age one would have looked like for Nora. Would she have been walking or crawling by then? Babbling or talking? Do one-year-olds even talk? I didn't know. And it was that not knowing but knowing I should that caused the sugar cookie in my hand to lose its sweetness as the toddlers' laughter echoed in my ears.

When I was young, a few years older than the boys busy before me, I used to take the two sides of the three-pane medicine cabinet mirror above the sink in my grandparents' 1970s-style bathroom and pull them into a small triangle. My skinny six-year-old self could barely fit through the large prism I made with the mirror. But once inside, there were endless images of me going on for miles in many directions, in what I imagined as multiple worlds.

Maybe if I ran to it and looked into that same magical mirror, it would show me what life might have looked like with a brown-haired little girl, born between these two boys, following along as she chased them on her own wobbly one-year-old feet. But no matter how hard I hoped, I couldn't envision it.

All I could see was Nora as a breathless newborn, eternally stuck in a sliver of time while her cousins toddled around joyfully, dodging the piles of presents for them under the tree with no topper. These beautiful beings would grow. Their bodies, thankfully, would morph in form as they aged from baby, to boy, to awkward adolescent, and ultimately into adulthood.

Nora was stuck forever at the age of "never born."

chapter 33

MOTHER BUT NOT

The traffic light turned from red to green. I pushed down on the gas pedal and the car's hum radiated through the sole of my shoe. Andrea, my fellow bereaved writer friend I met online, sat next to me in the passenger seat. Her eyes sparkled bright as she spoke about her daughter, who also died too soon. The last thing I saw before hearing the sound of metal crushing against the oncoming car was her brushing her short blond hair from her brow. Bracing my body with one arm against glass, the vehicle tilted. I frantically searched for Andrea, but she was gone, and again it was my fault. Unable to breathe, I reached for my belly before blackness abounded.

I jolted up in bed, adrenaline pumping. Georgie, who had been asleep between my legs, lifted his furry head. Realizing I was in my bedroom and not driving the car, I reached for my phone on the nightstand. Its bright screen boldly displayed the time: three a.m. The time I heard the words, "no heartbeat." My body remembered in my dreams that something tragic had happened exactly one year ago.

Recalling I was twenty-four weeks pregnant, I wrapped my hand around my midsection, searching for the baby's movements within me. She was silent and still. *Probably sleeping*, I hesitantly told myself, but I had to be sure. Pushing my fingers into my tight skin, I poked, forcing her to wake, needing to feel her flutters.

Holding my breath after a minute that seemed like months of no motion, she moved. Two and then three quick firm kicks. Sighing deeply, I cried whispered tears of relief but waited for seven more strong shifts that assured me she was alive.

With my eyes finally adjusting to the blackness of the room, I watched the rhythmic rising and falling of Nick's silhouetted chest as wetness wandered down my cheeks. Georgie, unsure of what to make of this after-midnight madness, moved from between my knees and up to the crown of my head, where he nuzzled his nose into the damp pillow next to my tears. Appreciating the act of empathy, I rubbed my face into his fur. An undeniable kick from baby number two, finally, totaled ten strong movements, different than that day a year ago when three soft shifts were all her sister had made.

Unable to fall back asleep, I headed to the kitchen for a glass of water. The crescent moon set outside the window, its dull glow barely breaking through a barrier of gray clouds. A year ago, I stood before that window in the glow of a fuller moon as Nora was dying inside of me.

Shivering at the memory, I walked back up the stairs to sit in the recliner. The smell of last night's smoldering coals rose as dawn's sunrise slowly burned away the moonbeams. Soon after, Nick woke and got ready for work. Respecting his wishes of not wanting to stay home with me and his sorrow, I kissed him goodbye before he went out the door and into the wicked winter landscape that blew in a familiar chill.

After Nick left, I sat down again on the recliner, this time with my laptop and the intention to write, but my hands started to shake. To ground myself, I stared at the inches of snow that piled high on the porch railing outside the window, glistening in the morning sun. The bulk of my pregnant belly suddenly became burdensome as my heart beat wildly. Feeling once more like I had followed a rabbit down a deep dark well, I squeezed my eyes shut, fighting my body that was bringing back the intense grief.

According to the experts in trauma and grief, this is exactly what happens around death's anniversary. Your body remembers. *The Body Keeps the Score* is the title of well-known psychiatrist Bessel A. van der Kolk's book. That's why the scent of smoke, the chill in the air, the sheets of snow that met the sunrise, the morose moonlight, the nightmare, and the three a.m. waking felt so familiar. As the anniversary of Nora's stillbirth arrived, my body sensed the sameness in the scenery. The *feel* of that decisive day from a year ago, somehow had found its way into this one.

Breathing slowly and reclining back on the sofa chair, I calmed myself. Unable to find the words for my next *Knocked Up Blogger* post due to the editor in two days' time, how could I convey this conundrum of being a mother, but not, when pregnant with my second baby on the anniversary of the death of my first?

It was as if my motherhood spread between two unseen worlds of birth and death. Both daughters lingered in the land of nothingness that we go to when we die and come from when we are born. My children were invisible to others as they resided in this land of the unseen. Parenting two daughters, one only in memory and one in dreams to be but not one in the physical realm of reality. It's a strange way to mother.

My fingertips fiddled with the Nora footprint pendant around my neck. Needing a break from trying to type, I opened another tab on my browser and brought up Facebook to see if anyone had posted in the online event created to honor the day we should have been celebrating one year with Nora instead of acknowledging one without.

Because Nora means "light," I asked family members and friends to post photos of luminescence in the *Honoring Nora: Show Me the Light* closed Facebook group. The scrolling seemed endless.

Images of illumination filled my feed. Candle flames contrasted against darkness, sunsets strewn with pinks, purples, and blues above Nora's name handwritten in the sand, thousands of Chinese lanterns lifting into an ebony star-filled sky, and a rainbow-colored nebula bursting out of blackness in outer space, were hundreds of photos others posted to show me there was still light in the darkness . . . to show me my life was brightened by Nora.

Tears turned to sobs. My pain mingled with other people's love, bringing forth a broken beauty. Others in my community weren't as lucky. Their loved ones ignored their babies, denied their despair. But not us. A year later, strangers, family, and friends still sent love our way by acknowledging Nora's light. Angels were real; they dropped off casseroles and didn't shy away from speaking my dead child's name.

Putting my computer aside, I entered Nora's nursery and pulled out the decorative papier-mâché bird-covered box I had bought at the craft store. Inside the bin were the baby ballet shoes she never wore and the first story book she received from Grandma Barb, *Love You Forever* by Robert N. Munseh. When my mother-in-law gave it to me while pregnant with Nora, she said it was her favorite. Nostalgic tears appeared in her eyes, recalling how she used to read it to Nick nightly as a newborn.

Thumbing through the book, I read the refrain out loud, "I love you forever, I like you for always, as long as I'm living, my baby you'll be." It was a love song written from a father to his two stillborn babies, I would later learn. A love song I now understood.

Putting the book down, my attention turned to the items on top of her dresser, gifts for Nora given to us over the last year. A baby block with her name, weight, and one date branded into the wood. Handwritten notes and cards cluttered around the first photo of her—a black-and-white ultrasound profile print of Nora in my womb taken the day we named her. And the blood-stained pink knit hat she wore after her silent birth.

Item by item, with each memento placed into the burial-sized box, I began feeling a place within my body under the weight of grief, open for Nora and this new baby to be.

Taking a deep breath, I sighed as I surveyed the room. In what was once Nora's nursery, I had made space for her sister to maybe one day sleep inside. The only piece of Nora's memory that remained was not a memory at all but the ugly urn that held her ashes. Without thought, I reached for the tiny bronze box and placed it in the corner of the larger one. Closing the lid to the bin felt like closing a tiny casket. Everything I ever had of Nora I then placed on the top shelf of my closet next to my winter sweaters.

When Nick came home from work and passed by the nursery, he panicked. "Where is Nora?"

Leaning against the nursery door, I rested a hand on my belly. "I put her away."

"You what?" he asked sharply.

"I thought it was time."

Through pursed lips, Nick insisted, "Where is she?"

Surprised by his anger, I explained, "In our closet. In the memory box I bought—"

Nick brushed by me in the doorway and hurried toward our bedroom. His shoulders tightened as he rounded the corner into our closet. He found the box on the top shelf, flipped open the lid, and immediately took Nora out from the spot I had nuzzled her into earlier. Without words or eye contact, Nick walked by me and put Nora's urn on top of his dresser. Tears cut through my concealer at Nick's need for continued connection to his daughter.

Later that night, Nick stood in the glow of the open refrigerator door and grabbed a handful of carrots. Still sullen, he ate them over the sink while looking away from me out the window. "Lindsey, come see this."

"See what?"

Our dark and frozen front lawn had become an illuminated snowy landscape. Over fifty golden flames fluttered inside white paper lanterns on the sidewalk in front of our home. Two shadowy figures in snowsuits, beanies, and boots floated, like angels, against a charcoal sky.

"It's the neighbors," Nick said, reaching for my hand as we watched silhouettes tromp back through hills of snow and into the house next door.

chapter 34

CHOOSING HOPE

January snow blanketed the landscape outside the window of Anna's office during another Friday morning therapy session. Small white flakes fell to the earth as if in a snow globe, like how they did the day before Nora died. The kind that isn't too cold and falls slowly from the sky, meandering down to the earth below, where it sits like cotton candy on the barren branches it rested upon. It reminded me, sadly, of the last time I believed in hope.

"What are you thinking about?" Anna interrupted my thoughts after closing her office door. She sat across from me on the couch parallel to the window framing the wintery scene.

Still gazing out the glass, I replied, "I was thinking about how I once innocently thought I would feel better after a year of grieving. In the early days of mourning, after the bricks of grief buried me and I had crawled out from underneath its weight, I thought grief would eventually leave as time moved forward." I smirked at her. "And that future me, a year from Nora's death, wouldn't still be sitting here, on her therapist's couch, complaining about her suffering."

I scoffed at the memory I kept to myself of innocent me in the forest when the snow dusted my shoulders and my warm arms wrapped around a newborn-sized Nora in my womb. Past me was so naive. She had no idea of what her life was about to become. If I could go back to that hike in the woods before Nora was stillborn, would I tell her what her future held?

Anna, with two fingers framing her face, nodded her empathy in my direction. "What does this suffering feel like now?"

Twiddling my thumbs in my lap, I said, "It feels like instead of leaving the bricks of grief that buried me behind, I gathered them up in a backpack and brought them with me."

Taking off her glasses, Anna held her teal-rimmed rectangle lenses in one hand with the stem end in her mouth.

"I mean I was so naive in my early days of grief, thinking I could project my way out of this pain."

Anna tapped the temple tip of her frames to the top of her lips. "What if your Grief Project was a way for you to exercise your grief muscle?"

"What's a 'grief muscle?'" I used air quotes that emphasized my suspiciousness of her answer.

She chuckled. "It's how some explain the grief process. Grief is described more like a muscle. Instead of believing that time heals all wounds. Over time, people learn how to hold the pain of grief. The weight of the original loss stays the same as time moves on, like you mentioned," she waved her hand, holding her glasses toward me, "with your brick backpack. But it's not the time, it's the bereaved, like you, who become stronger at carrying it." I nodded as she finished. "Your Grief Project was a wonderful way for you to *be* with your grief. To *surrender* to it. To continue to connect to Nora so deeply, which you still do."

"That makes sense," I said, while shifting positions in my seat to accommodate the ache in my side caused by my widening waistline.

Anna, nodding toward my soccer ball-sized, twenty-six-week belly, asked, "Have you been connecting to this baby?"

Shivering, a sense of shame skimmed my skin. To avoid answering, I looked out the window. Snow had accumulated into inches in less than an hour on the windowsill. Tears formed in the corners of my eyes, feeling warm against the air's coolness. "I want to connect, and I try, but I'm too scared. I connected last time." My voice cracked. "I had hoped last time, and everything was taken away."

Exhaling deeply, Anna placed her glasses back on the bridge of her nose. "I know you are really scared. I can see why being vulnerable and having hope is hard for you. What does Brené Brown say in her new book, *Daring Greatly?* Something like, 'Softening into the joyful moment of our lives requires vulnerability.' Connecting to this baby takes a great deal of it, which I know you struggle with. Especially after losing Nora." Anna collapsed her hands into a prayer pose in front of her lips. "But, Lindsey"—she swallowed hard—"what if this baby dies, too?"

Taken aback by her question, I froze and tightened my eyes into a squint, unsure if I was angry or aghast at Anna's audacity. "What are you saying?" I asked, sharply.

"I'm asking, how would you feel if you didn't connect to this baby like you did Nora?" She nodded again toward my middle, "And then this baby also died."

My stiff muscles melted at Anna's gentle delivery of such a harsh challenge. Running my right hand over my bump, I contemplated what I might be missing by continually being cautious about connecting to this baby. Or what this baby might be missing from me? I had been so focused on the broken bough of my last pregnancy that I inhibited myself from bonding with baby number two. "So, what do I do?"

"That's for you to decide." Anna's eyes moved from mine to the window, where a strip of sun peeked through the early morning snow shower. "But remember Lindsey, hope is a choice."

✒✒✒

That following week was the beginning of the third trimester, at almost twenty-eight weeks pregnant. We once again sat on the living room couch in front of the warm orange glow of another smoldering winter fire, where exactly a year ago from then we had spent our days in early grief. This time, though, we were attempting to choose hope, by choosing a name for Nora's sibling.

"What about Nicole?"

Nick shook his head, not taking his eyes off the television, binge-watching episodes of *Breaking Bad*.

"What about as a middle name?" I looked up from my phone where *What to Expect When You're Expecting: Top 100 Baby Girl Names* was pulled up in my browser. "It's the female version of your name."

Nick shrugged. "Maybe."

Frustrated in not finding the right fit for baby number two's name, I worried it might jinx this pregnancy. In some cultural traditions, giving a baby a name isn't even considered until after birth. Is that why Death arrived to take Nora, because we named her before she was born??

Scrolling through names on the screen as an act of defiance to my incessant fear about this baby's future, I had made it to the end of the alphabet and Nick had made his way to the end of another episode as the fire dwindled to red ambers. "What about the name Zoe? It means life."

Nick turned his full attention toward me with raised eyebrows. "I like it. Isn't that how your dad always addresses you in birthday cards and texts he sends you?"

"Yeah. Since I was in high school, he started calling me Zoe after he traveled to Greece for work one year. He thought I embodied the name."

When I was sixteen, my dad had handed me a gift from his

recent travels with my new name written on the envelope of the attached card. He had chosen my nickname because I was his "lively" daughter, with an insatiable zest for life. Strange how none of life felt like that anymore.

Nick grabbed my hand and flashed a hopeful smile before he said sincerely, "Then let's call this baby Zoe Nicole. She can be named after you and me."

chapter 35

I HAD TO
BELIEVE

The weeks passed slowly during the third trimester. The frigid
February winter with its negative twenty-degree temperatures showed no sign of leaving, just like my fear that something
might happen to this baby. But at thirty weeks pregnant, I continued attempting to choose hope about this pregnancy as Anna had
challenged me to do, and this time doing so by balancing on a stool
in the nursery to hang white letters of Zoe's name above a crib
designated for her sister. Knowing that my bump would only grow
bigger and not yet feeling the clumsiness that comes at full term,
the balancing act on the stool was much easier than the daily one
of balancing hope and fear I clumsily carried as we inched toward
Zoe's due date at the end of that March.

With each day of this pregnancy, I learned how intertwined
the extremes of life's emotions were braided together. For every
act of hope we embraced, like naming Zoe, there was an equal
and opposite action made from fear. There were no birth classes
or buying baby clothes, still too afraid to jinx this baby's arrival by
preparing to bring her home.

Around thirty-one weeks pregnant, as another act of choosing
to hope, we had a photographer take our maternity photos, but

also hired a doula as a backup plan in case this baby also died at birth. We needed the extra support. Our doula, Natalie, was in her late thirties with long, thick, black hair that touched her tattoos covering both arms.

On a dark and damp sloshy February evening, she taught us about a C-section birth and helped us prepare for, hopefully, welcoming Zoe into the world.

The delicate dance of hope and fear only became more difficult as we entered week thirty-two of pregnancy. No longer were there weekly bump photos like in our past pregnancy, but instead we went to weekly nonstress tests, biophysical profiles, and prenatal appointments. My heart would pound, and my palms would sweat in the minutes before the sonographer placed the ultrasound wand on the skin of my round belly. Once I left these scans knowing my baby was okay, I would finally allow the tears of relief to flow, sobbing over my steering wheel in the parking garage of my provider's clinic before returning to work.

That week, in session, a client newly sober from an opioid addiction described to me her desperate need to chase another high, which led to her most recent relapse. With distracted focus, I laid my hands on top of my protruding belly and counted Zoe's kicks as I listened to my client list off her symptoms of irritability, insomnia, and withdrawal. That was when I realized how I, too, suffered from addiction, just a different kind.

Each time I would leave my doctor's office, I would find momentary relief from the devices that saw into the walls of my dangerous womb, but the release of fear only lasted a few hours before I needed another fix of reassurance from another appointment. I was reiterating to my client the coping skill of taking it one day at a time, which Alcoholics Anonymous preached, when I realized it was the same mantra I needed while going through this pregnancy.

But it was hard to remember this while asleep, where I couldn't escape fear in my dreams. For each evening brought with it a three a.m. waking. My subconscious remembered the exact time Nora had been declared dead, which jolted me awake. In the dark silence of the early winter morning, before attempting to fall back asleep in the same spot one baby died, I would lay on my side with my hand tucked under my tummy and between the mattress to steady my shakiness as I waited for my alive baby to move. Anxiously, I poked at her, forcing her to wake. In whispers to her sister, I closed my eyes and asked her to keep Zoe safe. In response, a subtle shift took place under my skin. Nora's voice accompanied Zoe's motions repeating, *Mom, you get to keep her.*

At the reassurance of movement, I exhaled. Two more shifts followed the first to make a total of three. Then another followed by what I envisioned was a forceful baby shoulder shrug. My child was already annoyed at me from within the womb for forcing her to wake. I knew I was putting my anxiety onto Zoe and worried what effect this may have on her. Like an addict, I couldn't stop. I needed to be certain she wasn't dead like her sister before I fell back asleep. I poked again on the side of my stomach that my anterior placenta did not cover. She wiggled, rolling away from my requests for reassurance . . . so different already than her sister.

At thirty-four weeks pregnant, Kristi nudged me toward hope once more by insisting on throwing me a mother blessing, as I wouldn't commit to another baby shower and avoided others. Instead of the guests engaging in the shower tradition of bringing gifts for the baby, during a mother blessing, inspired by the tradition of the Navajo ceremony of a blessing way, a woman's passage into motherhood was celebrated. Women who love the expecting mother bring their own birth stories, listen to her fears, and circle her in a sisterhood of support to send her off with a sense of hope for her child's birth.

Kristi, wearing a flowing teal and pink bird-print dress, arrived at my house early on the last Saturday afternoon in February to set up for the celebration. She decorated our dining room in colorful papier-mâché bird garlands and lit lemon-scented candles in our living room with aqua and pink ribbons that matched her outfit. Tags were fastened to the wax on two of the candles for both Nora and Zoe. Three other women besides my sister, who had walked with me while grieving, sat with me in a circle on my living room floor. After the first hour had been spent hennaing my round belly and guests' different body parts, we talked about births that ended in both life and death.

Kristi sat to my left and started the ceremony by lighting Nora and Zoe's designated candles. I watched with a smile as she sniffled, holding back tears, while reading from the back of the colorful card she had painted herself.

Kristi passed the task of sharing onto Claire, my bubbly bereaved mom friend who I met at Faith's Lodge. Seated next to my sister with her hands clasped beneath her chin and elbows on her knees, she shared her wishes for me. I listened closely to her warm words that resonated, as she, too, knew how hard this past year had been grieving one child while expecting another. A baby bump protruded underneath her black-and-blue striped maternity sweater.

Andrea, my bereaved mother mentor and fellow writing friend, went next in sharing her wisdom. She sat across from me, crisscross, in the circle of support. On her wrist, still drying, was the henna tattoo of her dead daughter's name. A few years ahead of me in her own grief journey, Andrea had served as a lighthouse for me in my mourning. She floated easily between feelings of sorrow to glimpses of giggles as she read from her small, leather-bound journal. From her living example, I saw a flash of how in the future, my life, like hers then, might be filled with more happy days than sad ones.

Sloane, my best friend from college, sat next to me on my right to close our circle of support. With her newly-cut black bangs and freshly-painted blue nails, she was the last to share her hopes for Zoe's birth. Not a bereaved mother, but a mother who solidly supported me in my sorrow. When her smoky-shadowed eyes caught my appreciative grin, I nodded back my love for her.

I wiped away tears as Kristi closed the circle by reading notes from my mother and friends from high school that couldn't make it through the winter weather because they lived too far away. With only a few moments left in the ceremony, before we planned on moving on to mingling, my friend Taylor, who I also met at Faith's Lodge, burst through the front door along with the blunt February breeze. Taylor held her three-month-old daughter, born after the death of her son, bundled up on her hip as she closed the door behind her.

"Sorry I'm late," Taylor said. Squeezing herself into the seat between Andrea and Claire, she set her baby, Margaret, who had rosy chubby cheeks and a matching polka-dot dress like her mother, down on a blanket spread out in the middle of our circle. Watching Margaret wiggle on the carpet, I was surprised that I was not annoyed or jealous that this baby with a blue bow in her wispy brown hair was there. Instead, it brought a little bit of hope into my heart.

"Did everyone already go?" Taylor asked, as she pulled out a piece of lined paper from her diaper bag. Unfolding it, she smoothed out the creases before she cleared her throat. "I've already been through this part of the journey," she said, as she looked at her daughter and the rest of us followed her gaze. Then her eyes settled on mine as she continued, "I know how scary it is to be you right now, Lindsey, because I was scared, too. The only advice I can give is that I had to believe. And now I just have to believe for you, and for baby Zoe, that she will come into this world alive." Her stare was serious but soft, as she repeated, "I just have to believe."

Appreciative, I smiled back at Taylor, but still struggled to believe this baby might live.

A week later, at thirty-five weeks pregnant, winter inched into March. A thick blanket of snow still covered the ground outside from the long winter, and I laid under a thick comforter in bed. Again, counting the minutes for Zoe to move as the sun rose, I found myself poking and prodding my belly. It's in the moments that she did not respond that I was certain she was dead. Flashbacks to the words, "no heartbeat," that marked her sister's demise flooded my mind. "Please, baby, move. Please." I was no longer asking but begging her to respond. Ten minutes went by without movement. Then fifteen. I got out of bed and into the shower in a trance. Knowing I needed to get to work but fearing I would be headed to the hospital to hear those awful words again instead.

After my shower, I dressed in maternity slacks and a sweater before I laid back down on the mattress one more time to see if Zoe was still alive inside of me. Placing a hand on my belly I waited for her to move while planning her funeral in my mind. *Would we even have a funeral? Is losing a second baby a "fooled me once shame on fate, fool me twice shame on me" kind of scenario?*

Kick. Kick. Jab.

With those wiggles, my chest heaved with uncontrollable sobs. "Thank you, Zoe. I love you so much! Please don't die!" burst from a place of deep love for her within me that I had pushed away throughout the entire pregnancy. Thankfully, a subconscious connection had still grown between us.

I whispered softly toward my belly, "I love you." Both hands wrapped around my middle, hugging Zoe from the outside of my womb.

I left for work but was distracted more than usual, going through the motions of seeing clients and feigning attunement to their needs with *hmms* and *uh-huhs*. In between each appointment, I would lie down on the couch, a cushion still warm from where a client just sat, and count Zoe's kicks to make sure she was still alive while I begged Nora to reassure me her sister would get to stay. Client after client, I attempted to hold their pain while I pushed down mine. After five therapy sessions of being distracted, I canceled the rest of my day and went home during the early afternoon.

Walking through the garage door into the house, I dropped my winter coat and boots onto the entrance rug and rushed up the steps. I passed Nick, who was reading a book on the sofa next to George and closed the door to our room, where I threw myself onto my bed once more.

"What's wrong?" Nick asked, peeking in from the cracked door where he found me weeping into the same pillow I had wept into earlier that morning. He made his way from the outside of our room onto the edge of our bed, where he sat next to me in his sweatpants and sweatshirt. With my back turned to his, he brushed my hair as I sobbed. "I can't do this any longer. It's so hard, and I'm so tired." I looked over my shoulder to face him. "This morning, I thought she was dead!" My nostrils flared as I started to hyperventilate.

"Slow down. Just breathe." Nick moved his body closer to mine, creating a spoon shape on the bed.

"I want this to be over!" I wasn't just speaking about that morning. I was recalling all of it. My chest heaved. Nick pulled me closer to him, and I heard him sniffle. I felt like Shell Silverstein's *Giving Tree*, with no leaf, apple, branch, or trunk left to give. Everything I had, I'd already used up to get this far.

"I'm so tired of missing Nora and making sure Zoe doesn't die, too." Every day I carried around one life in the passenger seat of my womb, where the last person who sat there died, and I could never take a break from being the driver, worried this car might crash again.

I continued crying into the pillow soaked with my tears, but my breathing slowly became more regular as Nick held me. "How do we do this?" Lying face-to-face, I felt his warm billowy breath against my wet cheeks. "Love this much, knowing we can lose it all again?"

Nick stroked a strand of hair away from my forehead and then let his fingers follow the frame of my face, cupping my chin gently in his hand. He repeated Taylor's words from a few days before. "We just have to believe."

I looked down at my belly and placed my hands on top of Zoe inside of me, begging for a third time my same whispered wish. "Please stay."

chapter 36

A DIFFERENT BABY, A DIFFERENT STORY

"Lindsey, you talk about fear, but I hear more sadness in your voice. Is there sadness?"

Tears flowed again as Anna asked this question in our therapy session on a sunny but gray sky morning in mid-March, nine days before Zoe's scheduled birth.

"Yes. Sadness is there. But I'm also confused." I wiped away my tears, leaving mascara marks on the tissue. "All I know of birth is death. And as Zoe's due date approaches, I fear that when I deliver her, the journey of being a parent will be over again."

Anna flashed an empathetic smile across her freckled face before glancing at the wall clock above my head. I assumed we were running late on time, but she continued. "It makes sense that you feel that way. But what if it's different this time, and baby Zoe lives?"

My stomach fluttered, and it wasn't Zoe kicking. "Honestly, I haven't allowed myself to think about anything past her birth."

"But it does sound like you're starting to think about it." Anna spoke in her whispered, always kind, fairy godmother tone. "The leaps of faith you've already been taking to bond with Zoe . . . if you can do that, I think you have the strength to consider how you might feel when you bring her home."

"I don't know." Feeling defeated, I wished she could sprinkle some pixie dust on me and magically, a breathing baby Zoe would appear in my arms.

Leaning back in her bright-orange chair, Anna intruded upon my fantasy with practicality. "How do you plan on getting through the next week and a half?"

"I have no idea." I was like a deer in headlights on a desolate highway as Zoe's birth approached, paralyzed by fear. I wasn't sure if I should jump out of the way of the oncoming car, run toward it head on, or just wait for it hopefully to safely pass me by.

Anna glanced at the clock again, but this time said, "It's time to go."

I grabbed my winter jacket and we both stood from our seats. Anna walked to the door, and I waddled. Before she opened it, she said, "I'll be thinking of you."

"Thanks," I replied, "It means a lot, no matter what happens."

"Well, I'm here. No matter what happens. But I believe the next time I see you; I'll also get to meet baby Zoe." Anna winked before she shut her office door.

The weekend after my therapy session and five days before my scheduled C-section, I sat quietly in the passenger seat of the car as Nick and I ran last-minute errands before Zoe's planned birth. On the way home from the grocery store, we waited for the traffic light to turn from red to green in front of the brown-bricked crematorium where Nora was last whole. We had been stuck in this liminal loop of becoming parents for almost two years.

"Do you think it will be different this time?" I asked Nick, while I watched the black roofs of houses blur together.

Nick moved one hand off the steering wheel to take mine on top of my once-again watermelon-sized belly. "I hope so," he said tenderly.

Outside, specks of mossy grass tried to reach up to the spring sun through melted patches of dirt-stained snow. Taking a deep breath, I inhaled the aroma of a wet earth beginning to bloom again. "I hope so, too. Anna asked me if I had thought about what it will be like if Zoe lives and had we prepared to bring her home." I spoke to his profile as he watched the road. "And you know what? I don't think I have." Subconsciously I shook my head. "I feel unprepared for what it might be like. I know a healthy baby is what we have wanted for the past two years, but I don't think I've allowed myself to think about what we need to do if that happens. I think that is what Anna was getting at. And now I'm nervous that we haven't done anything to prepare. Is that strange?"

"No. That makes sense. What can we do then?"

"I'm not sure. When I think about doing anything for Zoe past her birth, it reminds me of how Nora never came home." The image of us cheerfully naming Nora after our first ultrasound flashed through my mind.

"With Nora, we were so ready in every way. Remember how awful it was to put all the new and never-used baby stuff back in storage? Makes me sick to my stomach. I don't want to go through all that again . . . I can't go through that again."

Taking his eyes off the road to connect with mine for a millisecond he asked, "I know you haven't wanted to prepare. But Linds, maybe it's time to start?"

Nodding, I rubbed the top of my belly underneath my fleece jacket. Maybe I needed to take one last leap of faith before this baby was born. Noticing the big box stores we just drove past, I asked, "Can we make one more stop? I have an idea."

That evening, Nick and I stood in the nursery rummaging through a drawer of clothes designated for Nora that she never wore, which we hoped Zoe would. We struggled to pick out socks in the right shade of pink to match Zoe's coming-home outfit that we had spontaneously bought earlier that afternoon.

In a moment of courage, we stopped at Babies "R" Us. Walking among breast pumps, bottles, and complicated, adjustable strollers, we searched for an outfit for Zoe that would be just hers. We settled on a polka-dot rose-pink and teal onesie with a matching hat and mittens. It now hung by a hanger on the handle of the nursery's dresser. The newborn outfit symbolized so much. It was as if I had been holding my breath since I saw the positive pregnancy test nine months ago and that I wouldn't exhale until Zoe took her first inhale.

We stared at the tiny baby outfit. With a sound of uncertainty in his voice, Nick said, "It seems real now."

"Yeah," I replied, with a sound of trepidation in mine. We had just completed the tasks of indifferently packing a hospital bag and reluctantly bringing baby furniture out of storage. Going through the motions of checking off items on the to-do list of preparing for this baby, I was reminded of how we had done all these things before, but last time with more joy and excitement. I wrapped both arms around the outside of my belly with Zoe inside, recalling how I once did the same in the days before her sister's birth.

"It just seems like pregnancy is the main event. It's hard to imagine bringing home a baby," Nick continued, without taking his eyes off the polka-dotted onesie, which represented a long-held wish.

"I know. I hope it happens," I whispered, while standing next to a changing table once again expectantly filled with wet wipes and size one diapers.

Nick reached for my hand. Our fingers interlaced and firmly locked with the other before he replied, "I hope so, too."

birth

"You are my sunshine,

You make me happy when skies are gray . . ."

—*Jimmie Davies, "You Are My Sunshine"*

chapter 37

GIVING BIRTH
TO LIFE

"What time is it?" Nick groggily asked, half asleep. The glow from the bathroom light flooding the darkness had woken him as I stepped into the bedroom after taking a long shower.

"It's four a.m." I squeezed into my maternity leggings and sweater one last time. Pulling at the bottom of my shirt to cover the skin of my stomach that peeked out I added, "I couldn't sleep."

I hadn't slept since three a.m. when I always woke up, spending the twilight hours before Zoe's birth tossing and turning, constantly waiting for her to move within my waterbed womb. I had whispered an altered version of the old bedtime prayer my mother had my sister and I recite each night. "Now I lay me down to sleep, I pray that Zoe I can keep. If she should die before I wake, I pray to the Lord my soul to also take." This mantra monopolized my mind in the hours before morning's sunrise.

"Do you mind if we go to the hospital early?" I asked Nick, still sideways under the sheets.

He threw the covers off to the side and stepped out of bed to take a shower.

Waiting for Nick, I nervously and hesitantly checked and rechecked the hospital bag to make sure everything we needed was packed. Toothbrushes, deodorant, nonmaternity leggings and a shirt for me, an extra shirt and pants for Nick, and Zoe's polka-dot outfit were neatly folded and tucked inside the small suitcase. Nora's silver footprint pendant necklace in a small gray jewelry box sat on top of all the items.

Zipping the suitcase closed, the vibrations from the two sides of the zipper came together as the two emotional sides of this journey of grief and joy also intertwined. When the top of the zipper reached the end of its path, a twinge of hope floated into my heart that pushed away the last nine months of fear. Like Anna in *Frozen*, it felt like the first time in forever I could believe again in hope. "Could you put the car seat in the car before we leave?"

Zipping up his sweatshirt that he wore to Nora's birth, he asked, "Are you sure?"

I had sworn to myself for the last nine months I was not going to blindly put my trust back in fate by taking a car seat to the hospital, with its lonesome straps and light weight, but something shifted and finally seemed right about having hope.

Nick brought the car seat up from the basement before putting it and the hospital bag in the trunk of the car. When I once again walked past an expecting nursery, I didn't close its door this time.

Nick drove right instead of left, taking the back roads toward the city instead of the interstate of last time. The radio was off, not on like it was the time before, and in the silence, I searched for the missing moon in the sky. During the drive, my hands never lingered from Zoe inside my swollen stomach. "Move, baby girl. Show me you're there," I whispered, as I waited for her to respond.

"I felt her!" I yelled a little louder than I had intended, breaking the quiet in the car. "She just moved again." Nick had driven over a pothole, which must have jostled her awake.

"Good! Keep kicking little girl," Nick cheered, as he reached for one of my hands resting on my mountainous middle, where Zoe continued to wiggle.

My wish I made to the universe over the last two years was about to come true.

Once at the hospital, I sat on a bed in a paper-thin blue surgical gown, hooked up to a fetal monitor that found a heartbeat. The *flub flub* of Zoe's beating heart boomed like a drum over the machine's speakers. Relieved, I smiled wide as I waited to be taken back to surgery, while a tear dripped down Nick's cheek. "What's wrong?" I asked gently.

"Nothing. It's just really . . . *happening*."

With a hairnet lining my eyes, I looked lovingly at him and silently said, "Yeah, it is."

"Ready?" one of the two nurses standing in the doorway asked before entering the room. Nodding back at them, they both helped me up. We left Nick and Natalie, our doula, in the pre-op room, where they changed into scrubs for surgery while the nurses walked me down the hall.

The double doors to the operating room opened, and a coolness gushed through my smock. The blinding sterile lights hit my eyes hard, and the antiseptic stench invaded my nose. A reflexive response to squint and gag created a queasy feeling in my stomach. I hadn't thought about the possible risks to my body during birth but seeing masked-covered faces of medical professionals, and hearing the beep from their machines made anxious goosebumps prick my skin.

Buttressing my bare bottom against a cold metal cot, I faced the almond-shaped eyes of the calm nurse who encouraged me to breathe as the anesthesiologist poked my spine with an epidural. After turning me over, the medical staff swabbed my swollen middle with antiseptic and draped a clean blue paper covering over me, vertical to my neckline, separating my body from my head, which seemed apropos, as that is how I felt. By the time the numbing agent started to work below my waist, every part of me trembled above my breastbone. The horrible shaking in the present brought me back to the shivers of the past when the fever and infection stole Nora from me in the night.

Willing myself away from memories already made, I focused on the touch of Nick's hand on my cheek after he and Natalie had entered the room. Nick's concerned eyes locked with mine behind his own accessories of a surgical mask and hairnet. Bending over to take his father-he-hoped-to-be seat by my side on a stool near my head, I saw the silver footprint pendant dangle free around his neck from under his blue scrubs. "Lindsey, I'm here."

"I didn't recognize you behind the new outfit," I joked, flashing him a nervous smile.

Our brief conversation was then interrupted by my doctor who announced, "Here we go."

"You got this!" Natalie cheered, patting my shoulder with one hand as she held a camera in her other. She peeked over the curtain as the surgery began, while Nick's face was next to mine so he wouldn't see the incision.

Overwhelmed by hearing my heart pulsing in my ears, I moved my focus onto the surgical lamp above my body. In its reflection, I watched as the doctor lacerated open my abdomen and wiped away blood that bubbled out of my middle. I didn't wince at the sight of the yellow iodine antiseptic mingling with the crimson red color oozing out of me or the pull I felt at my pelvis because within what seemed like seconds of the incision, I heard a sound I'd waited years to hear. A sound that was eerily absent at our last birth. The most sacred sound. The screaming of my second daughter gasping for her first breath.

And with her wail, I saw her wrinkled face and her white, ver-
nix caseosa-covered body in the cylindrical surgical lamp above
me. She flailed her arms wide, moving her legs and screaming
loudly. But I didn't say, "Hush little baby," because I needed her
to keen . . . to cry for her, for me, for her sister she would never
meet, and for defying Death.

She was *alive!*

I had given birth to life. And this time, Death and her long
shadow were absent from the room. Instead, the sound of clapping
and *oohing* abounded as the nurses cheered for our breathing baby.
The doctor raised her up in the air in a sense of triumph for everyone in the operating room to see.

"Is she okay? Is she okay?" I repeated a hundred more times as
Nick broke his smitten stare at our second daughter and leaned in
to kiss my lips. His wet tears rolled down the side of his nose and
then dropped onto my face, mixing with mine. "Yes. She's okay!"

Monitors continued beeping and buzzing as our baby was
handed to the nurses at the warming station. Three of them tossed
her back and forth like a football over the scale, weighing, wiping, and finally wrapping her in a receiving blanket. Natalie gently
tapped Nick on the shoulder, nudging him toward our newborn in
the warmer. I stared at him, staring at her in disbelief.

"Can I touch her?" he asked the nurses.

"Of course!" They laughed and placed our breathing baby in
his arms for the first time.

Nick carried our newborn with a gentleness only a bereaved
dad would have across the operating room and toward me supine
on the surgical table. "Is she okay?"

"She's perfect!" Nick said, placing our baby on my chest.

When the weight of her little bundled body touched my bare
breast, a piece of my heart forever melted and the hole in my
soul that was missing Nora deepened a little. "She's so warm," I

uttered in disbelief that this baby was not cool to the touch like her sister.

Disoriented by grief and how the past could show up in the present, I searched our newborn's face for a person who was not there, hoping for a moment I was meeting Nora once more. The dissociation only lasted a second. Within Zoe's next breath, my soul filled with an indescribable love for her.

She was a beautiful baby, with long reddish-brown eyelashes, and big pink lips. The color of her eyes were deep blue, and when she opened them and they met mine, my heart whispered *thank you* to whatever and whoever was out there listening, to be able to keep this new little bundle of life we had created.

"We did it!" I said to Nick, as Zoe laid on my breast between our gazes. He smiled back, brushing away a hair on my brow that had escaped my hairnet. Bending down, he kissed my lips again as I held our warm, breathing baby, Zoe.

"Yes, we did," Nick replied through relief-filled tears. "And she is beautiful, just like her sister."

chapter 38

A CAR SEAT

"Is this baby Zoe?" A doctor wearing a white coat covering his tucked-in shirt and tie asked, waking me from a short slumber. The bald-on-top pediatrician stood over Zoe's bassinet. He unwrapped her from her blanket where she slept and placed his stethoscope on her chest. We had been in the hospital for a few days and were looking forward to going home. We just had to wait for the pediatrician to complete Zoe's final checkup.

"Yes," I said through new mother exhaustion. Rubbing my eyes, I rolled over on the bed and heard a soft squeak sputter from Zoe's mouth when the coolness of the scope met her skin.

"Good," he replied, as he threw his stethoscope over his shoulders, letting it hang around his neck. He swaddled Zoe back in her blanket and bent down to pick her up. "Baby Zoe and you will be going home today!"

"Really?" I sat straight up, suddenly wide awake, "Are you sure?"

"Yup. Tell your husband to get the car seat. It's time to go." He handed off a fussy-but-cozy Zoe into my arms. "Congratulations. I've heard you've had a long journey."

Nodding, I met his empathetic gaze. "Yes, we have." He nodded back with a gentle grin before leaving the room.

Carefully standing, making sure to mind my C-section stitches, I carried a bundled baby over to the room's rocking chair where I shushed her subtle squawks by swaying her back to sleep. My toes moved the chair from front to back and back to front as I studied her soft face and ran my fingertips over her wispy, strawberry-blond hair, not chocolate like her sister's. My own mother's melody of "You Are My Sunshine," came to mind, and I sang a modified version that I once sang to Nick. "You are my Zoe, my only Zoe. Please don't take my Zoe away."

Whispering into her ear between sniffles, I pleaded the magical words that worked through her pregnancy, hoping they would still work now that she was here. "Please stay." Cuddling her warm body close to my chest, I worried she might not wake, even though I could feel her breath rise and fall in rhythm with my rocking. Would the nine months of worry ever go away. But does a mother's fear about her child's future ever subside? The answer must be no.

A mother's love is as wide as the ocean and worry rides on top of its waves as the tides of life come and go.

Before I had time to ruminate any longer, Nick returned to the room with a cup of hot coffee in his hand.

"We get to go home!" I blurted out in a hushed tone before he could complete the kiss he bent down and placed on Zoe's forehead and then mine.

"We do?"

"The doctor stopped by and said we are good to go."

"Great! I'll start packing up her things." Nick placed his cup on the counter next to the sink and our makeshift sanitation station, where a breast pump and bottle parts used overnight sat out to dry. He hurried around the room, filling two large totes like a passenger packing who was running late for a flight. Each bag was brimming with gifts our family and friends had dropped off, along with extra diapers and wipes the staff insisted we take home. Nick nonchalantly slipped the purple, not blue file folder into one of the bags, and I made a mental note that the folder was full of a different kind of discharge paperwork this time than the time before.

"I'm going to take this stuff to the car. I'll be right back." His arms overflowed with so many items I didn't know a baby needed that he had to do a little dad dance of juggling his daughter's two large totes with his wife's duffle bag. He struggled to reach for his keys sitting next to his cup on the counter.

"I'll have to come back for the coffee," he teased.

"You mean, you'll have to come back for us," I said, smiling.

"Yeah. That's what I meant." He winked with arms full as he jostled through the door.

Ten minutes later, Nick returned with one arm hooked under the pink polka-dot car seat intended for Nora. Staring at it, I reflexively reached for Nora's necklace I had put back on, along with my going-home clothes, while Nick took our things to the car. Silently, I clutched the pendant that held my dead daughter's tiny footprint. The nurse unbundled my living daughter from her wrap, nudging me to hold a naked Zoe she placed in my arms to bathe.

We never bathed or dressed Nora ourselves. It was too hard to consider. We abdicated the duty to the nurse. We didn't get to do so many things with her, I thought as I placed Zoe into the water where she screamed at its touch. I didn't mind, even though it was obvious Zoe did, for squawks were sounds we never heard from Nora.

We dressed a freshly-washed and soapy-scented settled Zoe in her pink-and-blue polka-dot newborn outfit and posed for a going-home picture as a family of four, but only three that could be seen.

"Make sure you get one you like," the nurse who held Nick's phone insisted. I bounced Zoe against my breast and looked over the nurse's shoulder at the photo she was wanting me to approve. A lightness of relief radiated from my face in the picture and almost lifted away the darkness of worry I had been wearing every day for the last nine months. I hadn't worn a grin that great in over a year.

It really does get better, but not in the way you think. Your life and heart grow bigger to hold both loss and love.

When I looked closer at the photo glowing from the phone, I saw my smile did not wash away the subtle sadness that had settled into the creases around my eyes.

The grief never goes away. The place inside you where you carry it becomes deeper, bigger, and wider for you to hold it, like a family that outgrows their home and moves into a new one so everyone can have their own room. You make room for grief and the one you're missing. We would always make room for Nora.

"Thank you," I nodded. "It captures everything."

Nick wrestled and nestled Zoe into her car seat. His hands fumbled over the straps and buckle. We both were new to this phase of parenthood. After we heard the buckle snap, Nick slipped one arm through the handle of the car seat, full with the weight of a healthy child, and smiled wider than I believe he did on our wedding day. Flashing my own smirk back at him, I reached for Nick's free hand, and the three of us walked out the double doors of the maternity ward and into the hospital hall.

Passing an elevator before the exit to the parking garage, I remembered fifteen months prior when we stood next to the fortunate couple gushing over their breathing baby girl as they stepped onto the elevator. My eyes settled onto Zoe snuggled into a car seat under a pink blanket tucked below her chin, just like the fortunate couple's baby was that day over a year ago. Finally, we were that lucky family.

Holding onto the memory, I squeezed Nick's hand. "How does it feel to be walking out of the hospital with a baby this time?"

Nick slowed down his steps and then stopped right before the exit to the parking ramp. His large smile shimmered on his stubbled face. "It feels wonderful! I'm the happiest I've ever been. How about you?"

"It feels *so* good." A single drop of grief and another of relief released down my cheek, for the journey had been so arduous and long. Knowing what I didn't know fifteen months ago when I saw that happy-go-lucky first-time family was that maybe there was more to their story. Maybe when we witnessed them leaving the hospital on New Year's Eve, they were like us, leaving the hospital right then. Not a first-time family, but a family who after months or years of pregnancy loss, got to bring home their baby for the first time.

I leaned in and kissed Nick as he held the door to the garage with his back. We walked through the exit as parents with a full car seat in hand, making our way toward home with our breathing baby girl, and a somewhat sutured heart.

chapter 39

SOMEONE
LIKE YOU

On an April afternoon, sunshine peeked through the gray clouds when I brought Zoe to a therapy session to meet Anna. Carrying Zoe in her car seat up the office building stairs, she felt heavier than she did when we left the hospital. Three weeks after her birth, she was now the same size and age, if corrected for gestation, as Nora was when she was stillborn. A blanket my sister had made for Nora had her name embroidered on the bottom corner in bright-orange thread and was tucked tightly around Zoe's chin. The thin layer of cloth kept out the remnants of the cold winter that straggled in the air, even though spring had started to bring with it warmer winds.

Anna opened her office door with a smile that was as wide as her new, thick, bright-red-rimmed glasses. "Oh, there she is!" Her voice went high pitched and babyish as she squished her face closer to Zoe's. "Everyone is *so* happy you are here."

I took a seat on the client couch with Zoe settled into my arms while Anna sat down in her therapist chair. "How are you?"

Pausing for a moment, I breathed in Zoe's sweetness. Her long delicate fingers with almond-shaped nails like her sisters wrapped around mine. "It's so surreal, almost magical, to be sitting here with a breathing baby in my arms."

"I bet it is."

Zoe's bright-blue eyes closed, and she shifted into sleep as I told Anna the story of her birth and the experience of bringing her home that I still had a hard time putting into words. I talked about adjusting to the difficulties of breastfeeding and the challenges of sleepless nights that I swore I would never complain about but did. *And* how I was beyond grateful for every day I got to keep Zoe, who lay in my lap, audibly tooting in her sleep, which made both Anna and I laugh.

I admitted to Anna it wasn't all magically better now that Zoe was here. The fears didn't go away overnight as I had hoped. I spent hours out of my evenings checking to make sure Zoe was breathing, counting her breaths.

"That is postpartum anxiety, and it could take time for you to recover," Anna informed me.

Which is why I would continue to work with her for another two years.

Chewing the inside of my cheek, I found the courage to ask Anna, again, the question I feared the most and even more now that Zoe was here. "I worry that I will forget her. That somehow while raising Zoe, memories of Nora will fade away."

I didn't dare add the line out loud, *along with my love for her.* Instead, I looked at Zoe's cherub face while clutching the Nora hand-print necklace around my neck. "You see, it's getting harder for me to remember her now. The demands of raising a living child take away from the time there is to mourn a dead one. Dinners need to be made, chores need to be done, diapers need to be changed. The act of living goes on. With so much to do, it's easy to forget her." A single tear fell from my eye. "Not intentionally, but slowly, over time, I'm afraid she will slip silently away into the background of life."

"I've never lost a child, Lindsey. But I do believe that a love this great is never forgotten."

At Anna's answer, silent sniffles escaped my attempt at suppressing their release. Not wanting to wake Zoe, I whisked away tears with the back of my wrist. Noticing the little hand on the wall clock about to align with the big one, I composed myself and used the last moments of the session to express my gratitude. "Thank you," I told Anna. "I couldn't have done it without you."

Her eyes went soft, filling with a glow. "I am honored to have played a part."

Placing Zoe back in her car seat, I tucked the blanket intended for her sister around her stomach and stood from the couch to leave. Anna and I moved to the door together, ready to say our goodbyes when like other clients of mine often do, I left with a doorknob statement, only revealing my true vulnerability in the last thirty seconds of the session. "You know, one day I hope to help others like you do." Over my shoulder I looked around her office at the gray client couch with its brightly colored yellow pillows and her hip-orange therapist chair before I asked, "Do you think I could someday become a therapist for bereaved moms like myself?"

Anna held steady my questioning gaze. "I think you'd make a great grief therapist."

"*Hmm*," I lifted my shoulders to my ears, the heavy car seat in my hands went up and down with my shrug. "Who knows. Maybe one day I'll even write a book."

She nodded with a grin that grew behind her glasses. "I have no doubt you will." She then waved goodbye before closing her office door.

That evening after my therapy session, I took a shower before bed. As the steam rose and the water droplets formed into fog on the glass, I ritually carved the letters of Nora's name out of the dew upon the door. Four letters, short and sweet, like her life was, appeared on the windowpane, every morning and every night, because I placed them there. While the water from the shower head beaded off my back, I decorated her name on the glass with hearts and retraced the lettering over and over, taking a moment to remember her, if only for a minute so that I could be with her once more.

After my shower, propped up against pillows, I cradled a slumbering Zoe in my arms. A single tear slipped from my face onto Zoe's soft cheeks, as I held her in the same spot in bed where Nora had died over fifteen months ago. Van Morrison's "Someone Like You," played from my phone's speaker. Smiling sweetly in my second daughter's direction, I swayed as I sang along with Morrison's lyrics that seemed to parallel the hard road we had walked through the darkness after losing Nora. My voice cracked with each note of the song that played, and a wave of heat crept up from my scarred heart before I burst into tears, snot, and tremors.

I tried to gulp back my agony to not wake Zoe, but as I held her, I finally felt some sense of relief that mixed with a deeper grief I didn't know was still inside of me.

Nick must have heard me trying to repress my cries because he quietly walked into the room and over to where I rocked back and forth on the bed, cradling a still-snoring Zoe to my chest. Gently, he placed his lips upon my forehead. I averted my eyes from his, embarrassed by my gushing grief. Upon completion of his kiss, he let his cheek rest upon my brow and simply said, "Nora."

And with her name said out loud I nodded, eyes tightly clenched, as I continued crying. Behind my eyelids, it was as if I could almost see Nora again through the darkness.

Nick laid one hand on Zoe's honey-scented head and stroked her hair, while his other rested on the small of my back when he whispered into my ear, "I miss her, too." And with the warmth of his soft breath left upon the nape of my neck, I burst into one of the loudest, most forceful, most moving cries my body had yet experienced since the day Nora had died. It was as if grief was leaving me and deepening within me all in the same moment.

"Someone Like You," our wedding song, continued playing softly over the speaker as I gazed at our beautiful baby. My heart continued to break when I realized this deepening of grief was due to understanding that I would never get to have a moment like this with Nora. I would never get to hold someone exactly like her again. Every new memory I made with Zoe was a memory that I would never have the chance to make with Nora. The widening of this woe in my heart would forever grow as the days, weeks, and years of a life with Zoe moved forward and Nora's life would be left behind, standing still in its sliver of time, as we raised not Nora but someone exactly like Zoe, who brightened our darker days.

present

"You are my sunshine, my only sunshine.

You make me happy when skies are gray

You'll never know, dear, how much I love you

Please don't take my sunshine away."

—*Jimmie Davis, "You Are My Sunshine"*

chapter 40

EPILOGUE: EVERYTHING HAPPENS FOR NO REASON AT ALL

"You had another sister once," Nick's lullaby began.
Listening in from the hospital bed next to where he sat in a rocking chair, I stayed silent with my eyes closed, as he shared our family story with our brand-new baby boy. Nick and I had made the decision a year earlier that we wanted to give Zoe a sibling she could see and that our hearts could hold enough hope to make it through a second subsequent pregnancy. Born in May, Liev arrived three and half years after his first sister, Nora.

In what Nick thought was a stolen exchange between father and son, he breathed in Liev's newborn baby scent of sugared milk and possibility, before whispering into his ear, "Nora was her name. We loved her very much, just like we love you." The sound of his tears caught in his throat before he finished. "She didn't get to stay."

Opening my eyes, the afternoon spring sun spilled in from the window of the postpartum recovery room, illuminating Liev's little face. Pregnancy with him was different from with Zoe. I didn't hear Nora's voice guiding me through, like she did with his sister.

And fear, my faithful friend, still visited, but less often, which was probably why the birth of my third baby felt like closure to the chapter in my book about creating life within my womb.

Our son slept wrapped in his pink-and-blue striped receiving blanket snuggled in Nick's arms. Nick said Nora's name out loud for the first time in a long time.

It makes sense he would start our last child's story where our first's ended. Parents meeting their baby for the first time, quietly together post-delivery, where all of life was supposed to be ahead of you and not behind. Our son seemed to understand the hidden message in the tragically beautiful lullaby his father sang to him. *We're all connected. Even to the ones that never lived.* His story, starting with her ending.

Nick continued speaking gently to our little Liev, about Nora, and recalled his love for her. How he held her like he was holding him. How he loved his daughter who died, missed her, and in the same breath was so glad that he—her brother—born in the wide wake of her little life was here, just like his second oldest sister Zoe. Both not replacing his love for Nora, but to love them separately, uniquely, and in their own way as he had learned, like I had.

Love expands with each new person we welcome into our lives. Like the universe, love is infinite.

Through a tearful smile I broke their moment by whispering, "I love you for loving them."

Five months later, on a warm autumn weekend, Zoe, age two, and Liev, a baby, played on the family handprint quilt stretched out on the living room floor that Georgie had also flopped upon. *Made with Love by Grandma* was inscribed into the delicately stitched tag sewn into the corner of the expansive blanket my mother-in-law had made.

"Where is Mommy's hand?" Zoe giggled as she jumped between the twelve squares of the quilt, like hopscotch on the sidewalk. She understood that a beloved's name was in the middle of each square, represented by a needlepoint silhouette of a handprint. "Tis one?" Zoe asked and pointed to the specific section her chubby toddler feet fell upon. Liev, with drool dripping from his chin, watched in delight as his sister played a combination of indoor hopscotch mixed with twenty questions.

Zoe made her way to the tiny hand in the middle square. Recognizing the familiar letters of her name but unable to recite them, she pointed to the pastel purple handprint and looked up at me. "Tis mine?"

I nodded back in agreement, not having the heart and her lacking the words to understand that it was a tracing of her dead sister's hand, used in place of hers, as the quilt was made for Zoe before she was born.

Moving her gaze toward a handprint the same size and shape adjacent to hers, Zoe tilted her wispy head of hair and inquired, "Tis mine, too?" This second tiny outline of a hand had her sister's name under it. "No, honey. That is sister Nora's handprint."

"*Oooh*," Zoe cooed. Her eyebrows raised as she nodded, as if implying she already knew.

And in some way, she might have. We talked to Zoe about Nora. That she had an older sister who died before she was born, not wanting to hide death from her, for she was conceived in its grief. This reality of her being born out of the place where death once lived bothered me more than her. Carrying with me a secret fear that remnants of my worries from that mournful pregnancy with her might have seeped into her soul while she was inside me.

Death's memory lingers long with the living it leaves behind. It did with me. Did it also with Zoe? Death left me to forever worry when her forehead got feverish that there may be a penance yet to be paid to Death for her life.

Having lost interest in the game of quilt hopscotch, Zoe made a beeline for the new door stopper that happened to be her sister's urn. Earlier in the day while the children napped, I grabbed Nora's ashes that still lived on top of Nick's dresser and placed her box in front of my bedroom door to keep the warm autumn wind from slamming it shut. In some way, I imagined that by placing her urn there, Nora was there, too, almost four years old.

Zoe squatted, her heels solid on the floor, as her toddler butt barely pressed against the carpet. She picked up Nora's urn and carried it into the living room. She then placed the ugly bronze box at eye level with Liev, who was attempting to crawl around the quilt. Some would witness Zoe's interaction with an urn as odd, even grim, but I found it endearing. Curious to see what she would do next and not wanting to lead the course of her actions, I tiptoed into the kitchen where I watched in wonder at my two youngest children interacting with my oldest, who only existed in particles within the time capsule between them. Not a moment of my motherhood hadn't been touched by mourning.

Motherhood was mourning. Nora's stillbirth made me forever a bereaved mother. But even when a child lived, there were parts of their lives that die as they age. The baby clothes that get packed away, the bottles and burp cloths no longer needed, and the once crib transformed into a toddler bed, were all brief phases of parenthood that leave as soon as they arrive.

"Never grow up." Some parents plaster in paint Peter Pan's words on the walls of their baby's nursery in response to this kind of grief, but as a bereaved parent I'd rather write, "Please, (I'm begging you), grow old," above their beds. Motherhood, like life after loss, was a constant balance of grief and joy.

Watching quietly from the confines of the kitchen, I listened patiently to see what Zoe would do next with Nora's urn. In quantum physics, it is said that by observing an object, you altered the state of said object.

I'm glad I didn't utter a word that would have interfered with what happened next.

Kneeling on the blanket, Zoe put her hand on top of her sister's small box between her and her brother and said, "Look, Liev!" pointing to the urn.

"Tis Nora. Sister Nora." She looked down at the little box and back at Liev who made eye contact first with Zoe and then with Nora's resting place. Why she did this, I'll never know, but it caused a mushy smile to arise on Liev's baby face, as if this was all normal for them both, having one living sibling and sharing one that was dead.

I guess, this was their normal, as it was the only kind of life they have ever lived. A life made possible by Death. Maybe, in some way that science wasn't yet certain of, both Zoe and Liev knew that a sibling came before them, dying in the place where they first lived. Maybe stored in their DNA, in their genetic roadmap to life, my children understood they were connected to another sister. They had shared the same womb, received the same blood, and floated in the same cells as they took turns residing inside me. Scientists have found that fetal cells cross the placenta and live on in a mother, possibly melding their genetic material with the damaged organs within their mother's body that need mending.

Maybe, the organ of mine that needed the most repair was my heavy heart and Nora's cells had been there all along, suturing its beautifully broken pieces back together. It resulted in us becoming a chimera on a microscopic scale. Scientists referred to this maternal child sharing of cells phenomenon as fetal microchimerism. Maybe that was why I could still feel her? It's even said that fetal cells from one baby could maybe carry over into the next. Maybe that was why my children seemed to sense her, too. But maybe—the biggest maybe of all—was that in the moments before we were born, we had a choice in the life we were about to embark on, and Nora chose to sacrifice her life so she could give them theirs. She made the decision no mother could ever make and left the gift of her siblings behind.

It would help if I believed all this. It even helped not knowing if I did. But I did know she was real. She did exist, even if just for a fleck of a second, in the grand scheme of time and space. And because of her brief existence, they existed, too.

I like to look at it as if our lives are nonlinear, with all our story-lines happening at the same time. It's only that our tiny human brains cannot comprehend the enormity of everything happening at once, so time and our stories somehow become sequential.

Einstein was said to have told a fellow grieving friend, "People like us, who believe in physics, know that the distinction between past, present, and future is only a stubbornly persistent illusion."[1]

This idea comforts me, even when believing everything happens for no reason at all, because it means all my children's lives have touched each other's. Their stories overlap and intermingle, even though all three will never hold hands.

In some ways, that was how their lives really were, like quilt pieces on opposite sides of the fabric, interwoven and linked but yet never touching each other's edges.

Liev would not be without Nora not being. His story begins years after hers and never had a chance at happening without hers ending. Zoe, in her exact form, wouldn't have been here either if Nora had lived. For the precise molecules of her makeup would have missed their moment to Big Bang together, bringing into being the girl we loved, with her stubborn will and sensitive smile. But maybe, in some version of this life, Zoe could have been, if Nora would have been, too. Nick and I had always planned to have a second child, making it easier to imagine that Zoe's existence could have slipped into this timeline, too. Her life did not have to depend on her sister's death like their brother's did.

Two, not three, was the number of children we had planned for, even if there was a time in our relationship where three was considered. In the early months of dating, on a warm summer's day, similar in sunlight to that afternoon my three children spent playing hopscotch on a quilt, Nick and I had cuddled on a hand-me-down-couch with torn cushions in his bachelor pad apartment. We talked about our separate dreams and compared to see if we were willing to entwine them like our fingers. Nick asked if I wanted kids and how many. I said yes and answered three. I thought there would be two biologically ours and one adopted. I never imagined having one dead and two alive. Maybe that was what the psychic I visited all those years ago saw. But years later, as I sat on our living room floor upon a made with love handprint quilt, that was exactly how our family shaped out to be. A girl, a boy, and an urn.

In two years' time, from our afternoon on the family quilt, when the smell of soil after yesterday's rainstorm lingered in the air, Zoe, Liev, and I played hopscotch again, but this time in our driveway sidestepping shrinking puddles.

Zoe asked, "Do wishes come true, Mama?"

I watched as my four-year-old girl brought the white fluff of a dandelion to her lips and blew the seeds of its skeleton into the sunny spring sky. Wondering how to answer, as parents did when struck suddenly with the task of figuring out how to break the cruel truths of life to our little ones without taking away all things magical and safe in the world.

If you would have asked me this question in the wake of Nora's death, I might have answered no, dreams were for the foolish and hope was an evil temptress. But now, with years of Zoe and her brother earthside hugging me in the morning and kissing me at night, each day reminding me that they were the miracles of light I fearfully and wonderfully made from a place of darkness, I realized I must give her an answer that's in between. One that encompassed the dialectic of life while being honest and simple, yet convincing enough for a preschooler to believe.

"Mama," she insisted, stomping her foot onto the pavement for emphasis of wanting an answer, "do wishes come true?"

"Well, you're here, and I wished for you." I smiled and brushed a stray strand of hair away from her heart-shaped face.

"Oh, how I wished for you," I muttered under my breath. Others may have wished for rainbows, for that was what they sometimes called babies born after one died, but my children born to me after birthing death were more like moonbeams, rays of light who illuminated the dark days of grief, making it easier to walk through the years in the "after" of loss, teaching me that death was not the central story—life is.

I searched for the moon in the daytime sky as Zoe patiently waited for me to be clearer in my response, for a child's curiosity was never completely satisfied with uncertainty. "Yes, sweetie. Some wishes do come true."

She smiled up toward me with childish delight as her belief in magic and miracles were confirmed. Her strawberry-blond hair, like mine, not dark-brown like her sister's, danced in the wind as she plucked from the ground another skeleton of a dandelion to make her wish upon.

"Good," she said, taking a deep breath and exhaling her wish into the ghost of a flower, "because I wished for Nora."

"Me, too." I sighed, witnessing tiny white wishes floating upon the breeze. A familiar warmth washed over me when I saw a single small sparrow fly away from the branch it was perched upon. Shivering, goosebumps appeared on my arms, even though the sun shone on my face. I sensed Nora making herself known to me through the tiny bird, through Zoe and her wishes, and through Liev, who just turned two, nudged Georgie, itching his collar, off the chalk hopscotch, as his sister searched for more potential wishes scattered along the sidewalk in front of our home.

It's not until now, years later, that I finally understand Elizabeth McCracken's ending to her memoir on stillbirth. "It's a happy life," and like she said, "Someone is missing," and always will be. Part of you never feels as if your family will ever be complete.

But for me, Nora is not fully lost. She lives on in the beams of light born after her, the beings that could not be without her not being. When I witness Zoe whisper her sister's name into the wind that carries away wishes, I see Nora has not left me completely, as I feared she might. For she is here not only in my memory, but in her siblings, too.

I watch Zoe's most recent wish be whisked away in the wind. Seeing her green eyes shimmer in the sunlight as her gaze follows her wishes into the air, I admit a truth to myself. Now knowing how this beautifully broken lullaby ends, I would choose to do it all over again, even if I couldn't change a note. For Nora's story is our story, and like love and lullabies, it lives on in our bittersweet ever after.

NOTES

INTRODUCTION

1. Nina Perry, "The Universal Language of Lullabies." BBC News. January 20, 2013.

2. Clare O'Callaghan, "Lullament: Lullaby and Lament Therapeutic Qualities Actualized Through Music Therapy." *American Journal of Hospice and Palliative Medicine.* 25(2): 93-99 (April-May 2008). doi:10.1177/1049909107310139. PMID 18198359 . S2CID 206633408.

Chapter 11: IT HAPPENED TO US

1. Elizabeth McCracken, *An Exact Replica of a Figment of My Imagination: A Memoir.* (Back Bay Books: 2010).

Chapter 30: A SIBLING, NOT A REPLACEMENT

1. Ünstündag -Budak, Ayse meltem. "The Replacement Child Syndrome Following Stillbirth: A Reconsideration". *Enfance.* No. 3 (March 2015): 351-364. doi:10.4074 /S0013754515003079. ISSN 0013-7545. S2CID 146133639.

Chapter 40: EPILOGUE: EVERYTHING HAPPENS FOR NO REASON AT ALL

1. Ira Flatrow, "Resetting the Theory of Time." Talk of the Nation. NPR, May 17, 2013, https://www.npr.org/2013/05/17/184775924/resetting-the-theory-of-time#: ~:text=Albert%20Einstein%20once%20wrote%3A%20People,that%20true %20reality%20is%20timeless.

ACKNOWLEDGMENTS

I n the early months of my mourning and into the dark years of my grief, it was the sisterhood of sorrowful mothers surrounding me with support who encouraged me to share my story. Other mourning mothers including Franchesca Cox, Lori Ennis, Rachel Whalen, Emily Long, Rachel Lewis, Jenny Albers, Kiley Hanish, Alexis Marie-Chute, and Dr. Jessica Zucker became my mentors by bravely sharing their own story of love for their child they longed for. It's because of them and fellow bereaved parents in the pregnancy and child loss community that this book came to be. To all named and not, I am forever beholden.

When you lose a baby during pregnancy or soon after, a subsequent community sprouts out of that place of darkness. That is why three months after my second daughter's birth, Pregnancy After Loss Support (PALS) was born, too. A place where grief and fear are held with hope. I'm deeply indebted to the PALS community, contributors, volunteers, donors, and board members that continue to make PALS possible. And I'm forever grateful for the most important member of our team, Valerie Meek—a virtual stranger who became my beloved friend, biggest cheerleader, and the heartbeat of PALS.

I've learned that books, like babies, don't come into being without a team to birth them. Thank you to Brooke Warner, Shannon Green, and the publishing team at She Writes Press who made my dream of becoming a published author come true.

Thank you also to Barret Briske for securing copyrights, Lorraine White and Cass Costa for editing my words, Maple Intersectionality Consulting for guiding me through a sensitivity read, and Lindsey Cleworth for designing a cover that captures the story, each assisting in birthing concept into creation. And I'm beyond grateful to Kate Hopper, my writing coach. A literary midwife. You stood by my side through years of labor as I birthed the lyrics to this lullaby into a book.

But it was Anna, my therapist, who helped me first find those lyrics to this lullaby by taking my hand in the darkness and guided me toward the light. You never asked me to choose between the two. I don't believe everything happens for a reason, but I'm so glad fate led me to find you. Not only did you hold sacred space for me in my mourning, but you also taught me how to be a better therapist. I appreciate both, deeply.

I'm lucky to be loved by my parents Bob and Gerry Fritsch, in-laws Paul and Barb Henke, Grandmother Debbie Fritsch, family members, and friends who always acknowledged and accepted my grief because they knew it to be love. I'm forever filled with gratitude to be loved so unconditionally, especially by my parents, who first taught me what love is.

Angels are real; they show up as sisters. Kristi Fritsch-Churan, you held space for a mother's grief even before you knew motherhood. Your sisterly love has always been more vulnerable and unlimited than mine. There are no words to convey my indebtedness to you except with a humble, thank you. I love you.

Words elude me when I speak of my undying love for Nick, my husband and best friend. But I hope the reader and you can find the words within this story. Our story. That you so graciously let me share with the world. Thank you for standing by me through the darkness. You never shy away from my broken pieces. You are the beginning of my love story, and I hope you will be there at its end. May we always hold hands in life until Death comes for us again.

As a skeptic of faith throughout this story, with its ending I found spirituality in motherhood. My spiritual teachers arrived as my children. Nora, thank you for making me a mother, showing me that love spans space and time. Zoe and Liev, thank you for bringing hope and joy back into my life, teaching me that a heart grows with every person you let in it to love.

And finally, thank you to Grief, my forever companion and reminder that I have loved at a depth that not even Death can extinguish.

ABOUT THE AUTHOR

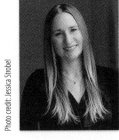

Photo credit: Jessica Strobel

Lindsey M. Henke is a licensed clinical social worker and psychotherapist specializing in the grief that accompanies life transitions. She founded Pregnancy After Loss Support (PALS), a nonprofit for parents pregnant after a previous perinatal loss or infant death. Her writing has been featured in the *TODAY Show*, *Pregnancy and Newborn Magazine*, the *Huffington Post*, and the *New York Times*.

Lindsey lives in Minneapolis, Minnesota, where during winter she can be found with her nose in a book. The rest of the year she enjoys hiking with her two living children and husband.

SELECTED TITLES FROM SHE WRITES PRESS

She Writes Press is an independent publishing company founded to serve women writers everywhere. Visit us at www.shewritespress.com.

Carry Me: Stories of Pregnancy Loss by Frieda Hoffman. $16.95, 978-1-64742-359-9. Finding little literature or support available after suffering two miscarriages, Frieda Hoffman decided to create the resource she wished she'd had—real stories about pregnancy loss from real women, free of the off-putting lenses of religion or academia—in the hopes that it will provide other women comfort and wisdom when they need it most.

Expecting Sunshine: A Journey of Grief, Healing, and Pregnancy after Loss by Alexis Marie Chute. $16.95, 978-1-63152-174-4. A mother's inspiring story of surviving pregnancy following the death of one of her children at birth.

From the Lake House: A Mother's Odyssey of Loss and Love by Kristen Rademacher. $16.95, 978-1-63152-866-8. When thirty-nine-year-old Kristen Rademacher loses her baby, she must endure the barren and disorienting days an aching mother faces without her child, accept the consequences of rash decisions and ill-fated relationships, and nurture a mysterious healing that takes root while rebuilding a life and identity forever altered.

Hope is a Bright Star: A Mother's Memoir of Love, Loss, and Learning to Live Again by Faith Fuller Wilcox. $16.95, 978-1-64742-108-3. In this tender and honest recounting of her halting steps through the darkness of grief back toward the light of human connection after losing her young daughter to cancer, Wilcox offers compelling evidence of the redemptive power of love as a way to restore meaning to a world ruptured by loss.

I Know It In My Heart: Walking through Grief with a Child by Mary E. Plouffe. $16.95, 978-1-631522-00-0. Every child will experience loss; every adult wants to know how to help. Here, psychologist Mary E. Plouffe uses her own family's tragic loss to tell the story of childhood grief—its expression and its evolution—from ages three to fifteen.

Three Minus One: Parents' Stories of Love & Loss edited by Sean Hanish and Brooke Warner. $17.95, 978-1-938314-80-3. A collection of stories and artwork by parents who have suffered child loss that offers insight into this unique and devastating experience.